Mindfulness in Medicine

Rajat Chand • Greg Sazima

Mindfulness in Medicine

A Comprehensive Guide for Healthcare Professionals

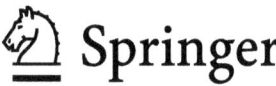

Rajat Chand
Diagnostic and Interventional Radiology
Austin Radiological Association
Austin, TX, USA

Greg Sazima
Senior Behavioral Faculty
Stanford-O'Connor Family Medicine
Residency Program
San Jose, CA, USA

ISBN 978-3-031-66165-5   ISBN 978-3-031-66166-2   (eBook)
https://doi.org/10.1007/978-3-031-66166-2

© The Editor(s) (if applicable) and The Author(s), under exclusive license to Springer Nature Switzerland AG 2024

This work is subject to copyright. All rights are solely and exclusively licensed by the Publisher, whether the whole or part of the material is concerned, specifically the rights of translation, reprinting, reuse of illustrations, recitation, broadcasting, reproduction on microfilms or in any other physical way, and transmission or information storage and retrieval, electronic adaptation, computer software, or by similar or dissimilar methodology now known or hereafter developed.

The use of general descriptive names, registered names, trademarks, service marks, etc. in this publication does not imply, even in the absence of a specific statement, that such names are exempt from the relevant protective laws and regulations and therefore free for general use.

The publisher, the authors and the editors are safe to assume that the advice and information in this book are believed to be true and accurate at the date of publication. Neither the publisher nor the authors or the editors give a warranty, expressed or implied, with respect to the material contained herein or for any errors or omissions that may have been made. The publisher remains neutral with regard to jurisdictional claims in published maps and institutional affiliations.

This Springer imprint is published by the registered company Springer Nature Switzerland AG
The registered company address is: Gewerbestrasse 11, 6330 Cham, Switzerland

If disposing of this product, please recycle the paper.

To our colleagues in healthcare, we offer this guide in gratitude for your tireless commitment, unwavering compassion, and selfless service.

Acknowledgments

Acknowledgment by Rajat Chand, MD, Austin, TX, USA

At the heart of my decision to embark upon the journey of medicine was a profound inspiration drawn from Osler's eloquent portrayal of "Equanimity" as the quintessence of the physician's character. This noble aspiration, coupled with an early and deeply instilled reverence for the supreme science of consciousness, set me on a path where I envisioned a profession that transcended mere occupation. I was captivated by the promise of engaging in a vocation where the battle against the palpable evils of disease was interwoven with the pursuit of groundbreaking scientific discoveries, all the while nurturing a journey of profound personal discovery. In this envisioned landscape, the practice of medicine emerged as the epitome of selfless action, a pure expression of helping others while detaching yourself to what matters less around you in such a setting, where every intervention and insight was detached from ego and dedicated to the greater good.

Yet, as I navigated through the corridors of contemporary healthcare, the stark contrast between the idealistic vision that drew me to medicine and the reality I encountered became painfully apparent. Far from being the sanctuary of supreme equality and wisdom I had imagined, the medical profession, as it stood, seemed to have been usurped by forces of ego, greed, power, and a pervasive disservice to the very beings it was meant to serve and imbue collegiality in. This divergence from the path of compassion and enlightenment was disheartening. The ancient texts discussing the science of consciousness, which led me on this path, with their dialogues on the profound desires to understand the essence of being, the universe, and the sacred cycle of life and death, seemed worlds apart from the US healthcare system's prevailing ethos.

Compelled by a desire to shield the unblemished optimism and potential for transformative change I saw in the eyes of those just beginning their medical odyssey, I felt an urgent call to action. My observations revealed we were perched on a precipice, where the choices we make could lead to a renaissance in healthcare or further entrench it in the quagmire of its present challenges. It was from this vantage point of critical introspection and hopeful vision for the future that the impetus to write this book was born.

The variety of teachings on consciousness, near synonymous with spiritual instruction in modern day, posit a universe where everything is connected and divine, advocating for a life of reverence towards all existence. They teach us that true liberation from suffering comes not from the external pursuit of material life but from the internal realization of our true nature, which many believe exists beyond the cycle of birth and death. This profound philosophy, emphasizing the purification of consciousness through the practice of meditation and unselfish action, seems to have been poised to integrate into the origin of healthcare and medical education, especially in a country like America, but also seems to have never gotten its foot in the door.

This profound integration appears to have been stymied, a curious omission in the evolution of a system deeply concerned with healing. To understand this conundrum, one must consider the historical and cultural milieu in which American healthcare and medical education blossomed. The inception and growth of these institutions occurred within a society profoundly influenced by Christian ethics and values. While Christianity, with its own rich tradition of contemplation and compassion, has undoubtedly contributed to the moral underpinnings of medicine in the West, its historically dogmatic stance towards alternative spiritual practices may have inadvertently erected barriers against the incorporation of meditation and consciousness exploration into medical education.

This exclusion can perhaps be traced back to a time when spirituality and science began to tread divergent paths, a bifurcation that became more pronounced with the Enlightenment and the rise of empirical science. The emphasis on rational thought and measurable outcomes, hallmarks of Western medicine's advancement, may have inadvertently sidelined the more introspective, experiential wisdom offered by practices like meditation. Such practices, rooted in the direct, subjective experience of consciousness, might have been viewed as antithetical to the burgeoning scientific methodologies that prized objectivity and reproducibility.

Moreover, the societal and institutional hesitancy to embrace these teachings could also stem from a broader reluctance to integrate what could be perceived as religious or esoteric practices into the secular and scientifically rigorous domain of medicine. This division reflects a broader cultural narrative that has often placed science and spirituality in opposition, a dichotomy that overlooks the potential for these realms to enrich and inform one another.

The oversight of not incorporating the teachings of consciousness into the heart of medical education represents a lost opportunity to foster a more holistic approach to healthcare—one that recognizes the inseparable connection between mind, body, and spirit. As we stand at the crossroads of healthcare's future, it is imperative to reconsider and potentially embrace these ancient wisdoms. By integrating the insights of meditation and consciousness studies into medical education and practice, we can cultivate a generation of healthcare professionals who are not only skilled in the science of healing but are also attuned to the multiple dimensions of wellness. Such an evolution would mark a return to a more integrated form of medicine, where the healing of the body is inseparable from the nurturing of the spirit, and where healthcare practitioners are as adept in tending to the inner landscapes of their patients and themselves, as they are in treating physical ailments. This reimagined approach could pave the way for a healthcare system that truly embodies the ideals of compassion, mindfulness, and holistic well-being.

Before I continue, it is important to acknowledge those who have supported me on this journey. To Dr. Shawn Sarin, for instilling the belief that perseverance sees us through to the end. To Dr. Karun Sharma, for emphasizing the universal humanity within us all. To Dr. Philip John, who never let me feel forgotten. Dr. Bairbre Connolly, for your invaluable mentorship and discipline. Dr. Dimitri Parra, for teaching the importance of mindful patient care and surgery. Dr. Dheeraj Gopireddy, whose work ethic and approach as a "Program Director" have been exemplary. To my parents, for teaching me the power of my words, thoughts, actions, and dreams, as well as the importance of spiritual progress. Dr. Alex Rhee, for pushing my boundaries and expanding my vision to the "bigger picture". Dr. George Koshy, for discussing tales of the Mahabharata on clinical rounds and always underlining the gravity of "Truth" in all that we do. Dr. Michael Temple, for shining in everyone's presence. Dr. Geogy Vatakencherry for instilling the utmost respect toward medical knowledge and patient care. And Dr. Joao Amaral, for demonstrating that kindness and courage are essential in medicine. Your collective wisdom and guidance have been indispensable.

Thank you to Margaret Moore and the team at Springer for supporting us in writing on this important topic. I must say, it took a lot of courage, so thank you for pushing us in this direction and giving us the opportunity to gain wisdom from the experience.

Last but not least, I must extend a profound acknowledgment to Dr. Greg Sazima for shedding invaluable education on this topic and serving as an ultimate guiding mentor. Our professional relationship, rooted in deep mutual respect and a shared passion for the betterment of healthcare, blossomed into a warm friendship for which I am forever grateful. His wisdom and guidance have been a lighthouse in the tumultuous sea of early career practice, illuminating purpose and the path forward with clarity and hardcore knowledge of the topic at hand. Dr. Sazima's mentorship has not only enriched my professional journey but has also left an indelible mark on my personal growth. For his unwavering support, insightful teachings, and the gift of his friendship, I am eternally thankful.

My journey through the medical profession, initially fueled by a quest for equanimity and the desire to serve, laid bare the chasm between the lofty ideals of mindfulness and compassion and the often harsh realities of medical education and practice. This book, then, is an attempt to weave in the timeless wisdom of the Vedic sciences, which has found itself into the foreground of our other most complex modern day sciences, offering a beacon of hope and a practical guide for restoring the soul of medicine.

This endeavor is not a call to eschew the scientific rigor that underpins medicine but rather to enrich our practice with a deeper, more holistic understanding of health and healing. It is not only a homage to my mentors, it is an invitation for all of us to contemplate how we might each contribute to a healthcare system that heals in the fullest sense of the word.

Acknowledgment by Greg Sazima, MD, San Jose, CA, USA

Wish fulfillment is an interesting, cryptic thing. Little wishes—to master a task, witness a great performance, visit a favored place—those are wonderful, but perhaps fleeting or trivial. The opportunity to fulfill a bigger, more potentially impactful wish that does not come along that often in our lives.

My own aspiration to master the concepts and fruits of this capacity of mindfulness had initially been in the "little wish" category, yet it has been immense to my own personal and professional life. To convey those same concepts and tactics in a broader way, to our patients and my peer professionals, is a bigger wish—and a privilege and an honor, too.

I so appreciate the fast friendship and easy working relationship with Dr. Rajat Chand, a compassionate and ambitious physician who generates in this aging doc an authentic optimism in the future of our calling. He approached me with energy and curiosity to work with him in shaping a guide that colleagues across our profession could rely upon. We are both hopeful that we've met that standard.

I would like to express my deep gratitude to all those who have contributed to my own understanding of mindfulness and its application in medicine. That starts with the collaboration of my work family of colleagues at the Stanford/O'Connor Family Medicine Residency Program, where we've taught and trained a generation of newbie docs in mindful medicine. Frances Respicio, LCSW, Katherine Mullins, MD, Michael Stevens, MD, and George Kent, MD, your support, wisdom, and encouragement over the years have been so valuable to me.

I am profoundly thankful to my own family—my lovely bride Tracy, and my sons Ryan, Matt, and Andy. Your support and understanding—and tolerance!—have allowed me the time and space to explore the exterior, tactical applications of this interior capacity and help formulate a guide that is user-friendly and accessible for colleagues across the ecosystem of healthcare.

I also extend heartfelt gratitude to my late mentor, Dan Jorgensen, and my friends and peers at Clear Mountain Wisdom, whose presence and collective support have shaped my understanding of mindfulness and its transformative properties, personally and clinically.

I am indebted to my patients who have generously shared personal stories and experiences with mindfulness. Your insights have added depth and authenticity to this book, and I am honored to have had the privilege of learning from your journeys.

My appreciation goes out to our team at Springer, including Margaret Moore and Henry Rogers, who worked tirelessly to bring this book to life. Your dedication to our project has been instrumental and much appreciated.

Last but not least, I extend my gratitude to you. Your interest in mindfulness and your willingness to explore its principles and practices are a testament to your commitment to the care of your patients—and your own well-being in a challenging job.

Thank you all for being a part of this mindful journey. May this book serve as a source of guidance and inspiration. Wishes can come true!

Contents

1	**Mindfulness in Medicine: Transforming Healthcare from Within**...	1
	Mindfulness and the Doctor/Patient Relationship	4
	Mindfulness and the Medical Office/Clinic	5
	Mindfulness and the Hospital/Healthcare System	6
	Mindfulness and Training Programs............................	7
	In Summary: Mindfulness for Medicine.........................	8
	Mindfulness 101	9
	The Science of Mindfulness	9
	Mindfulness in the Clinical Setting...........................	10
	The Mindful Healthcare Setting (Office, Clinic, Hospital, System, and Training Program)	10
	Mindfulness and Technology	10
	How to Use This Book	11
	References...	12
2	**Mindfulness 101**	13
	Mindfulness..	13
	Meditation...	15
	Setting Conditions...	17
	Learning How	18
	Applied/"Hybrid" Mindfulness................................	20
	Mindful Movement..	21
	Mindful Technology	22
	A Mindful Life Practice	23
	References...	25
3	**The Science of Mindfulness: Research and Benefits**	27
	The Roots of Mindfulness.....................................	28
	Systems and Networks	29
	The Limbic System and Mindfulness...........................	29
	Mindfulness, Neuroplasticity, and Neuromodulation	31
	Neural Networks and Mindfulness: DMN, SN, and CEN	33

	Brain Theory of Meditation	37
	Attentional Networks and Mindfulness	38
	Mindfulness and Improved Attention: Evidence	39
	The Impact of Mindfulness on Health	40
	Mindfulness and Pain	44
	Mindfulness Research: Future Directions	47
	Mindfulness: Research Limitations	48
	Mindfulness and Preventive Healthcare: Cultivating Resilience	50
	Mindfulness, Empathy, and Compassion	51
	Mindfulness and Acceptance	52
	In Summary: The Science of Mindfulness	53
	References	55
4	**Mindfulness in Clinical Care: Modalities**	59
	Learning and Teaching Basic Breath Meditation in the Clinical Setting: First, Ourselves	61
	Teaching Basic Breath Meditation: A Favored Approach	63
	The "Designated Sitter": An Office Mindfulness Liaison/Consultant/"Champion"	67
	Structured Programming	67
	Mindfulness-Informed Treatment Programs /Modalities	69
	Mindfulness-Based Stress Reduction (MBSR)	69
	Mindfulness-Based Pain Management (MBPM)	71
	Mindfulness-Based Cognitive Therapy (MBCT)	71
	Dialectical Behavior Therapy (DBT)	72
	Acceptance and Commitment Therapy (ACT)	73
	Mindfulness-Informed Treatment Programs /Modalities: Which One to Refer to?	74
	Resources for Mindfulness Training	75
	In Summary: A Wealth of Mindful Tools	76
	References	77
5	**Mindfulness in Clinical Care: Settings and Situations**	79
	Mindful Tools for Clinical Situations: Four Core Tactics	81
	The Office Visit	84
	Clinical Procedures	88
	The Mindful Medical Office: Implementation and Monitoring	91
	Implementing and Monitoring a Mindful Medical Office	92
	In Summary: Applying Mindfulness at the Bedside	92
6	**The Mindful Healthcare Professional**	95
	The Current State of Healthcare	96
	The Healthcare Professional's Temperament: Fulfillment and Risk	99
	Burnout	101
	Malpractice and Mindfulness	103

	In Summary: The Mindful Healthcare Professional	104
	References	106
7	**Mindfulness in Healthcare Teams**	109
	Those Were the Days	110
	Healthcare Teams and Stress	111
	Mindfulness and Healthcare Team Dynamics	113
	What Could Happen? Team Burnout	114
	Team... Mindfulness	116
	The Mindful Healthcare System	117
	Mindfulness and DEI	119
	Implementation	123
	In Conclusion: Real Team Mindfulness	124
	References	125
8	**Mindfulness in Healthcare Training**	127
	Mindfulness from the Start: Good for the Training, Good for the Trainee	128
	Mindfulness at the Outset of the Training Pathway	131
	Mindfulness Programming in Training: General Points	132
	Mindful Engagement in Educational Settings	133
	Mindfulness in Clinical Years (Residency, Internships)	134
	Mindfulness in Clinical Training Settings	136
	Voluntary or Compulsory?	137
	Sharpening the Message	138
	Mindfulness Training in Nursing and Allied Professional Programs	139
	Faculty Training	140
	Medical School Exemplar: Monash University School of Medicine, Melbourne	141
	Measuring Effectiveness	143
	In Summary: Mindful Medical Training	144
	References	146
9	**Mindful Technology**	147
	Technological Mindfulness	149
	First, We Can Sit	150
	"Bookending"	151
	Digital Diets and Detoxes	152
	AI: A Brief Summary of a Complex Topic	154
	Mindful... AI	155
	Mindful AI Technology for Patients	156
	Mindful AI Technology for Professionals	159
	Caveats	162
	In Summary: Mindfulness and Technology	164
	References	165

10 Conclusion: Mindfulness and the Future of Medicine 167
    Future Trends in Medicine: Advances and Concerns 169
    A Time to Act 171
    Finally, A Mindful Intention 172

Appendix A 175

Appendix B 181

Appendix C 187

Appendix D 193

Appendix E 217

Index 225

About the Authors

Rajat Chand, MD is a board-certified radiologist who is based in Austin, Texas. He specializes in both adult and pediatric diagnosis and intervention.

He has served as an author and editor for multiple textbooks, as well as a speaker for international medical conferences on topics related to both radiology and mindfulness.

Dr. Chand enjoys cooking, Brazilian jiu-jitsu, artistic exploration, and spending time with his pets. He will be a lifelong student in Yoga and aims to integrate eastern spirituality not only into his holistic view of healthcare, but also in teaching to future generations of physicians.

Greg Sazima, MD is a board-certified psychiatrist, educator, and author, based in Northern California. In addition to his psychotherapy practice, he serves as Senior Behavioral Faculty at the Stanford-O'Connor Family Medicine Residency Program in San Jose.

Dr. Sazima was born and raised in Cleveland, Ohio. He graduated in 1983 from the Johns Hopkins University with a BA in Social Relations; earned his MD in 1987 from the University of Cincinnati College of Medicine; and completed his psychiatric residency training at the University of Connecticut and Stanford University Medical Centers. He has maintained his private practice and teaching roles since 1991.

His current clinical, teaching, and writing/media work has included mindfulness and its applications in healthcare, the MD/patient relationship, and physician wellness. His first book, *Practical Mindfulness: A Physician's No-Nonsense Guide to Meditation for Beginners* (Turner Publishing) won the 2021 Gold Prize for Mind/Body/Mind/Spirit titles at the Foreword/Indies Book Awards competition. His essays on mental health and behavior have been published in the Sacramento Bee, Philadelphia Inquirer, and other periodicals. Volunteer work has included board positions at Capital Public Radio and Snowline Hospice.

Dr. Sazima resides in Granite Bay, CA with his wife, Tracy Brown Sazima, MD, a family physician in clinical and leadership roles at Kaiser Permanente in Northern California. The couple has three adult sons. Dr. Sazima has a deep interest in jazz piano yet only questionable skills in performance; his other interests include hiking, cooking, kayaking, and meditation.

Chapter 1
Mindfulness in Medicine: Transforming Healthcare from Within

There have been so many remarkable achievements in contemporary medical care. Advanced diagnostics and precision medical treatments continue to be developed for disorders across all of our specialties. Yet, the overall healthcare system has failed to deliver on its broader promise of high-quality, accessible, and affordable care. Despite the United States being one of the wealthiest and most technologically advanced countries in the world, our healthcare system is plagued by a multitude of thorny issues: rising costs, inadequate access to care, and uneven quality among them. Healthcare outcomes in the United States have been declining [1], with life expectancy decreasing for the first time in decades [2], and other measures of healthcare quality are also worsening.

Patients and healthcare providers alike are dissatisfied with the current system, with many feeling that the system is too complex, bureaucratic, and inefficient. The social, economic, and psychological stress generated by a world-historical pandemic has exemplified the best of medicine in just-in-time vaccines and treatments. But the blind spots in our system have been laid bare, especially in how we attend to the stress, trauma, and burnout so apparent in patients and treaters alike.

It's a paradox: both the best of times and the worst of times.

There are many factors that contribute to the paradoxical nature of healthcare today, and these factors can be interconnected and reinforcing. One of the key factors is the unequal access to healthcare, which can lead to disparities in health outcomes for different populations. This inequality can be driven by factors such as socioeconomic status, race, ethnicity, and geography.

Another factor is the profit motive that underpins much of the healthcare industry. While ideally industry-provided IT technologies supposedly free up physicians' time and energy for the human side of care, in practice the result is often ever-increasing productivity expectations that consume any time savings. These factors can create a paradoxical situation in which we healthcare providers are expected to deliver high-quality, patient-centered care within a system that is impacted by financial incentives and productivity targets. Burnout and disengagement among

© The Author(s), under exclusive license to Springer Nature
Switzerland AG 2024
R. Chand, G. Sazima, *Mindfulness in Medicine*,
https://doi.org/10.1007/978-3-031-66166-2_1

healthcare providers often results, as well as frustration and dissatisfaction among patients who feel that their care is not being prioritized.

Our patients have their own challenges in managing that dilemma.

Many individuals are poorly informed about best practices for their own self-care and may even be actively misinformed by unvetted, self-serving sources in the social media environment. The media ecosystem plays a significant role in shaping people's attitudes and behaviors toward their health. Unfortunately, much of the media content in this space is geared toward appealing to more primal consciousness targets, such as fear, grievance, and pleasure. This can manifest in ways such as priming people's fears about death and illness, amplifying controversies about public health recommendations, or promoting the "hidden-cost" pleasures of junk food and other unhealthy habits. The media landscape is flooded with myriad diets, supplements, and exercise protocols, often with conflicting advice and confusing messages.

This drama can leave many people feeling overwhelmed and anxious, or even numbed to the idea of self-help altogether. A term for this is "monkey mind," where individuals constantly and mindlessly chase after the latest trend, yet never feel satisfied or fulfilled. A lack of engagement in true preventive care can result, with many people only seeking medical attention when they are already experiencing significant health problems. This approach to healthcare is reactive rather than proactive/preemptive, with a focus on fixing pathology rather than incentivizing personal opportunity and responsibility for one's own better health. In many cases, healthcare providers are incentivized to treat illness rather than prevent it, with little emphasis placed on preventive care or patient education. This lack of emphasis on self-care and prevention can lead to worse health outcomes for patients and a higher cost of care for the healthcare system as a whole.

The challenges facing our healthcare system are just one aspect of a broader trend toward increasing stress and uncertainty in contemporary society. Climate change, political polarization, and the erosion of trust in institutions all contribute to a sense of unease and dislocation. One of the consequences of this environment is a loss of contentment and well-being, as people struggle to find meaning and purpose amidst the chaos. Indeed, a paradox of technological progress is that while it has the potential to bring people closer together and make our lives more convenient, it also carries the risk of dehumanizing us and diminishing our capacity for empathy and connection. We risk losing touch with our own intuition, creativity, and emotional intelligence. This dehumanization can manifest in many ways, from the way we communicate with one another (often through impersonal text messages or emails) to the way we relate to our own bodies and emotions (often suppressing or ignoring them). It can lead to a culture that prioritizes efficiency and productivity over care and compassion, which can have serious consequences for our health and well-being.

The larger issues of an uncertain world cannot be easily solved, but there are areas that we can address, such as the loss of connectedness in healthcare in the midst of a rapidly interconnected world. This paradox highlights the need for fundamental changes in the healthcare system, with a focus on addressing the root causes of the problem rather than just treating its symptoms. It calls for a shift toward a more patient-centered and value-based healthcare system, where quality, access, and affordability are prioritized over profit and bureaucratic quicksand.

Achieving this will require a collaborative effort from all stakeholders, including patients, providers, payers, and policymakers, to ensure that the system works for everyone. An essential part of the solution to this paradox can be found not in a new technology but in a very old one: mindfulness, cultivated through meditation.

While technology has made great strides in improving healthcare, it has also contributed to a kind of reductionism in healthcare, reducing complex medical problems into smaller, more manageable pieces. Yet this reductionism in healthcare has its downsides, often leading to an incomplete understanding of the patient's overall health and well-being. It can overlook the influence of and interplay among multiple factors, such as social determinants of health, environmental and inequity factors, and especially the mind-body connection. It can also lead to a distancing from our patients' emotional and psychological needs, inextricably linked with their physical needs. It similarly takes a toll on healthcare providers, causing us burnout, compassion fatigue, and a loss of meaning and purpose in our work (Table 1.1).

This reductionist tendency can mute empathy and dehumanize the truly human interaction. We can lose touch with the heart and soul of healing.

Table 1.1 The current landscape: A world increasingly interconnected yet experiencing a loss of connectedness in a reductionist model of healthcare

Reactive healthcare	The consequences	The implications
• Many seek medical help only when facing significant health issues, indicating a tendency toward a reactive approach • Lack of engagement in preventive care • Lack of incentivizing personal opportunity and responsibility for one's own better health	• **Poor health outcomes:** A lack of emphasis on self-care and prevention can lead to deteriorating health conditions • **Increased healthcare costs:** This approach results in higher costs for both individuals and the healthcare system	• **Neglect of preventive care:** This reactive mindset often leads to a disregard for preventive measures, increasing health risks • **Systemic bias:** Healthcare systems and providers often focus more on treating illness than preventing it, creating a cycle of pathology treatment over wellness promotion

Reductionism in Healthcare
- Simplifying complex medical issues into smaller parts often leads to a narrow understanding of overall health
- Inadequate Holistic Understanding: Overlooks the interplay of various factors like social determinants and the mind-body connection

Mindfulness, the trainable capacity of being present and nonjudgmentally aware of one's thoughts, feelings, and bodily sensations, has been shown to improve health outcomes, reduce stress and burnout among healthcare providers, and enhance patient satisfaction. Mindfulness-based practices such as meditation, yoga, and tai chi have been found to reduce anxiety, depression, and chronic pain, improving overall well-being. They have been shown to be effective in reducing stress, aiding in emotional regulation, and enhancing cognitive functioning. These benefits can have a positive impact on healthcare professionals, patients, and the healthcare system as a whole.

By incorporating mindfulness practices into healthcare settings, healthcare professionals can develop a greater sense of self-understanding and interconnectedness, which can lead to improved communication and collaboration with patients and colleagues. Patients can also benefit from mindfulness practices, as they can help them cope with the stress and uncertainty that often accompany illness and treatment.

Overall, while we may not be able to solve all the problems of an uncertain world, focusing on building self-understanding and interconnectedness through mindfulness practices can have a positive impact on healthcare and the people it serves.

The cultivation of our capacity for mindful awareness can and should serve as a heartful complement to our awesome technological tools. By incorporating mindfulness practices into their interactions with patients, healthcare professionals can create a more compassionate and effective healthcare environment that truly serves the needs of all individuals. Unfortunately, each realm of our healthcare ecosystem has its own particular, often paradoxical obstacles and challenges in truly incorporating mindfulness practices, starting at the source.

Mindfulness and the Doctor/Patient Relationship

For patients, whether wrestling with medical suffering or cultivating healthy self-care routines, mindfulness practices are clearly shown to be of benefit. Despite that scientific vetting, some patients may not trust meditation as a viable form of treatment. This may be due to misconceptions or preconceived notions about meditation—often around mystical or New Age tropes or perceived intrusions on the individual's own spiritual belief system. There may be a lack of understanding about "how it works"—how subjective, interior training can result in outward benefit. Many patients, often modeling the outlook of their physicians, may feel that medication or traditional psychotherapy is the only way to treat their conditions and may be hesitant to add complementary approaches.

It is nevertheless important for healthcare professionals to educate our patients about the benefits of meditation, and to encourage them to approach it with an open mind. Ironically, some physicians may not trust meditation as a legitimate aspect of treatment, even though it has been shown to be effective for a variety of health conditions. This may be due to our own lack of education about and understanding of mindfulness practices, or biases toward more traditional forms of treatment such as medication or surgery. Medical training curricula have traditionally been focused on the scientific understanding of the body and disease, which may leave little room for the exploration of complementary practices like mindfulness. Medical professionals often have demanding schedules, juggling long hours of patient care and administrative tasks. It leaves little room for us to explore new practices like mindfulness for our own self-care— even as we too could be optimal beneficiaries of these practices. The data to date and much of which we will highlight in this book show that medical professionals who practice mindfulness are more able to focus on patient care, better manage their own demanding workflows, and reduce burnout and compassion fatigue.

Our "see one, do one, teach one" custom applies here, in reverse: many physicians may be hesitant to recommend meditation to our patients because we have no personal experience in a meditation or other mindful practice. Without that direct experience, we are more likely to be ambivalent about its benefits, and unlikely to go further in learning how to incorporate it into our treatment plans with patients.

With both patient and treater walled off from working with mindfulness practices, the doctor–patient relationship can suffer. When healthcare professionals are distracted or rushed during appointments, we may miss important details or fail to fully understand our patient's needs. This can lead to misunderstandings, frustration, and a breakdown in communication between the two parties. When patients are less mindful and aware during their interactions with healthcare professionals, they may fail to fully communicate their concerns or ask important questions about their treatment plan. Patients may be more likely to experience anxiety or stress related to their healthcare experiences. They may become overwhelmed by the sheer volume of information they receive and feel disempowered in their interactions with us. This can lead to a lack of engagement with their treatment plan, missed opportunities to address their needs, and a lack of compliance. Ultimately, negative impacts on overall outcomes can result—for patients, healthcare professionals, and our relationships.

Mindfulness and the Medical Office/Clinic

Medical office staff have never been more stressed out. The demands of the work, amplified by the risks and routines of the recent global pandemic, have pushed many to leave the healthcare ecosystem completely. Managing multiple tasks at once, dealing with difficult patients or situations, and working long hours all contribute to the problem. Chronic stress has negative effects on both physical and mental health, leading to burnout, fatigue, and decreased job satisfaction. Like physicians, medical office staff may also experience compassion fatigue, becoming emotionally overwhelmed and exhausted from providing care to others. Feelings of cynicism, detachment, and reduced empathy toward our patients can often result. It is important for medical offices to prioritize the well-being of our staff and provide resources to help them manage stress, such as mindfulness practices, counseling services, and time off for self-care. By supporting the well-being of our staff, medical offices can improve the quality of care provided to patients and create a more positive work environment.

Nevertheless, incorporating mindfulness practices in a medical office or clinic setting can be challenging. Mindfulness practices emphasize nonjudgmental awareness and acceptance, which may not always align with the fast-paced, goal-oriented nature of medical work. Moreover, medical professionals often work long hours and deal with high-stress situations, which can make it difficult to find the time and energy to practice mindfulness consistently.

Another obstacle to incorporating mindfulness practices in a medical office is the culture of our profession. While we pride ourselves on our selflessness and dedication to caring for others, there can be a downside to this drive to prioritize the needs of others over some attention to our own well-being. Pressured to work long hours and take on heavy workloads, we can model this in our expectations for our staff and employees, toward sacrificing their own self-care and personal time. Moreover, the culture of selflessness in medicine may discourage medical professionals from seeking help for our own stress, reinforcing it as a sign of weakness or distraction from the mission. Modeling these distortions can lead to a culture of silence and avoidance around stress and mental health issues, impeding our natural mutual care for our colleagues, and negatively reinforcing the value of getting the help they need.

To overcome these obstacles, medical professionals can better educate ourselves about the benefits of mindfulness practices and emphasize their relevance to improving patient care. That begins with physicians recognizing and modeling the value of self-care and prioritizing our own well-being. Medical offices can build on that intention, creating a supportive environment that encourages self-care and provides resources for patients and staff to manage stress and mental health concerns, including mindfulness practices. A medical practice with streamlined mindfulness initiatives would even coordinate, monitor, and track such practices. This approach would create a sense of community and accountability and can make it easier for employees to incorporate mindfulness into their own daily routines. By valuing the well-being of all partners in care, we can improve the quality of clinical care provided to patients and contribute to a healthier, more sustainable healthcare system.

Mindfulness and the Hospital/Healthcare System

Widening the aperture, the same stress dynamics of needs, benefits, and barriers can be seen in larger healthcare systems. Healthcare is a high-pressure, high-stress field by nature, and it can be challenging to create a work environment that supports staff well-being. Research clearly indicates that healthcare professionals experience higher levels of burnout than workers in many other fields, and this can have negative effects not just on our well-being but also on patient care and outcomes. Most systems have recognized the importance of stress management for healthcare professionals and have been taking steps to improve the well-being of their staff. Addressing workplace stress requires a systemic approach, involving changes to policies, practices, and culture. This can be difficult to achieve in a large organization; there may be resistance to change among staff and leadership. Additionally, many healthcare systems face financial constraints and may not have the resources to invest in programs and initiatives to address stress and burnout.

Developing cost-effective, accessible, and customizable resources that systems can provide as part of their commitment to workplace health could help close this gap in cultivating a system-wide approach to mindfulness. Mindfulness practices can also be a valuable complement to DEI (Diversity, Equity, Inclusion) programming in the workplace. As an example, by providing access to guided meditations that address implicit bias and promote empathy for marginalized groups, employees can gain a deeper understanding of the impact of assumptions and implicit bias in the workplace. This approach can help to create a safe and inclusive workplace culture that values diversity and promotes a sense of inclusivity, empathy, and belonging for all employees.

One prime target in those systems that can have a force multiplying effect is in our medical, nursing, and other healthcare training programs, to begin that cultivation at the outset of healthcare careers.

Mindfulness and Training Programs

The teaching of mindfulness practices in medical, nursing, and other healthcare training programs is an obvious strategy. Healthcare professionals in training can develop a broader, more resilient foundation in emotional regulation, empathy, and communication—all part of our mission to provide patient-centered care. Medical training can be intense and demanding, and cultivating mindfulness can help students to manage their stress levels and prevent burnout. By learning mindfulness techniques, medical students can develop skills for managing stress that they can carry with them throughout their careers.

Even as mindfulness practices gradually become better recognized and appreciated as mainstream, secular tactics in self-care, healthcare educators, especially older faculty members in training programs, may not have a deep understanding or interest in mindfulness practices. This can be due to a variety of factors, including differences in cultural and generational perspectives, as well as personal attitudes and beliefs about mindfulness. Addressing this issue may include respectfully teaching some "new tricks" to those of us older canines, while accepting that some may not be interested.

But our mostly younger trainees are often more socially and culturally aware of the mainstream benefits of mindfulness practices. They deserve and in many cases are expecting a program culture that supports mindfulness and other self-care practices, and the resources and prioritized time for this as a part of their overall training. Ultimately, the most effective approach to teaching mindfulness in medical training programs will depend on a variety of factors, including the specific needs and preferences of students and faculty members, as well as the resources available to the training program. However, by incorporating a range of didactic, group-based, and online/app-based approaches, medical training programs can provide a comprehensive and effective mindfulness training experience for students, one that can produce valuable and real-time metrics.

Finding room in an already packed schedule of education and care is a challenge for physician faculty leadership. But by doing so, medical training programs can help to foster a culture of mindful care as well as support the health and well-being of our early career healthcare professionals who are our future successors in the "mission" (Tables 1.2 and 1.3).

Table 1.2 The path forward

Encouraging open-mindedness	Incorporating mindfulness in training
Educating patients about meditation's benefits and encouraging an open approach	Integrating mindfulness into medical training and professional development
Mindfulness in the medical office/clinic	**Mindfulness in hospitals and healthcare systems**
<ul><li>**Current challenges:** High stress, burnout, compassion fatigue among medical office staff</li><li>**Cultural barriers:** Perceptions of selflessness in medicine leading to neglect of self-care</li><li>**Strategic implementation:** Educating on mindfulness benefits, creating supportive environments, and incorporating mindfulness practices for staff</li></ul>	<ul><li>**Systemic stress dynamics:** High-pressure work environments leading to burnout and negative patient outcomes</li><li>**Systemic approach required:** Policy changes, cultural shifts, and investment in stress management programs</li><li>**DEI and mindfulness:** Incorporating mindfulness in DEI initiatives to foster empathy and inclusivity</li></ul>

Table 1.3 Mindfulness in training programs

Resilience building in trainees	Teaching mindfulness to healthcare professionals in training for better emotional regulation and empathy
Generational and cultural challenges	Addressing varying attitudes and beliefs about mindfulness among educators
Integrative teaching approaches	Utilizing didactic, group-based, and online resources for comprehensive mindfulness training

In Summary: Mindfulness for Medicine

The paradox of medicine at our current inflection point will not be easily resolved. In embracing and prioritizing mindfulness and integrating it into healthcare delivery from the consulting room through to the boardroom (and bedroom), healthcare providers can improve their own well-being and provide better quality care to our patients, leading to a more fulfilling and effective healthcare system for everyone.

As the title suggests, this book aims to introduce healthcare providers to mindfulness as it can be fostered throughout the medical ecosystem. Our audience of partners is broad and inclusive: our physician colleagues, other healthcare professionals, and healthcare executives.

- For physicians and other healthcare professionals, we offer insights into how mindfulness practices can help manage the demands of our jobs and enhance our communication and collaboration with patients and colleagues. It could also provide guidance on how to incorporate mindfulness practices into our work with patients and how to create a more mindful healthcare environment.
- For healthcare executives, we provide a framework for creating a more mindful healthcare organization, with a focus on promoting the well-being of both patients and healthcare professionals. It could also offer insights into how mindfulness practices can improve organizational performance and patient outcomes.

- For healthcare educators, we provide guidance on how to incorporate mindfulness practices into the curriculum for students and trainees. We highlight the importance of developing a culture of mindfulness within every training program and healthcare organization. Educational leaders play a critical role in shaping the education and training of future healthcare providers, so incorporating mindfulness practices into medical training programs could have a lasting impact on the healthcare system as a whole. By emphasizing the value of self-understanding and interconnectedness, leaders in medical training programs can help create a more supportive and resilient healthcare workforce.

Overall, we aim to bridge the gap between healthcare providers and patients by emphasizing the importance of building self-understanding and interconnectedness in healthcare provision. By doing so, we can help create a healthcare system that is better equipped to meet the challenges of an uncertain world.

The blueprint will include these successive areas of inquiry:

Mindfulness 101

- Concepts and definitions of mindfulness: a trainable capacity of mind.
- Types of mindful practices: formal (meditation, mindful movement), informal.
- Benefits of mindfulness: somatic, emotional, mental, social/interactive, spiritual.
- Basic breath meditation: an introductory guide with routines, tips, troubleshooting.
- Guided and manualized meditation approaches: a summary of current mindfulness-based therapies (CBT/CPT, Mindfulness-based Self-Compassion, Acceptance, and Commitment Therapy); a role for AI in individualizing guided mindfulness practices.

The Science of Mindfulness

- Understanding the Brain and Emotions: neural mechanisms behind mindfulness; the role of emotions in the brain; and the impacts of mindfulness on brain plasticity, neuroendocrine function, and immune function.
- The Impact of Mindfulness on Health: research on benefits of mindfulness in physical health conditions (cardiovascular disease, chronic pain, diabetes, cancer, and auto-immune spectrum disorders) and mental health (stress, depression, anxiety disorders, PTSD, and substance abuse).
- Current Research and Evidence: research on mindfulness and its effectiveness in healthcare, including the types of studies conducted (randomized controlled trials, observational studies); evidence supporting mindfulness-based interventions for different populations (cancer patients, veterans, and healthcare professionals).

Mindfulness in the Clinical Setting

- How mindfulness can be incorporated into clinical practice (consultations and medical procedures).
- The range of patient populations (medical, mental health) that benefit and matching them to mindfulness techniques that have been found to be most effective for each population.
- Training and support for medical professionals who want to incorporate mindfulness into their clinical patient care.
- Monitoring and evaluation of the effectiveness of a mindfulness program for patient care.

The Mindful Healthcare Setting (Office, Clinic, Hospital, System, and Training Program)

- Mindfulness for caregivers: the benefit of individual mindfulness programming for healthcare professionals.
- Mindfulness in Medical Teams: the benefits of mindfulness for medical teams in offices and clinics, including improved communication and collaboration.
- The Mindful System: overview of current projects in cultivating mindfulness in larger settings (hospitals, systems), planning, preparation, implementation, and monitoring.
- Mindfulness in Medical Education: how mindfulness can be used to improve the education and training of medical students and residents, nursing students, and trainees in allied healthcare programs.

Mindfulness and Technology

- Concepts and tactics in optimizing our own prudent use of technology in our work and personal lives, as well as identifying risks in use.
- Opportunities in using AI to overcome limitations in current/traditional mindfulness training and programming.
- The potential of streamlining mindfulness app-based programs (customization of unique individual experience, streamlining content, increasing accessibility) uniquely for healthcare organizations and training programs.
- Ensuring the philosophical foundations of mindfulness are integrated into the development of technology and that ethical considerations around its use (potential for bias, over-reliance, or misuse) are addressed.

How to Use This Book

As you embark on the journey through this comprehensive guide to integrating mindfulness into the multifaceted world of healthcare, it's essential to approach this book not just as a source of information but also as a practical roadmap for transformation. Whether you are a healthcare professional, executive, educator, or student in the medical field, this book is designed to be a versatile tool in your hands. Here's how to make the most of it:

- Understand the Foundations: Begin with the "Mindfulness 101" chapter to build a solid understanding of the basic concepts and practices of mindfulness. This foundation is crucial for both newcomers and those familiar with mindfulness, as it sets the tone for its application in medical settings. If you have never attempted a routinized meditation regimen, alongside this book would be a great place to start!
- Dive into the Science: The chapters detailing the science behind mindfulness and its effects on health provide an evidence-based approach. These sections are particularly useful for those who seek a deeper understanding of how mindfulness works from a neurobiological and psychological perspective. They will equip you with the language that you need to discuss mindfulness in more concrete scientific terms.
- Contextualize Mindfulness in Healthcare Settings: As you progress through the chapters focusing on clinical care, healthcare teams, and medical training, try to envision how mindfulness can be integrated into your specific environment each page of the way. Take notes every time you have this visualization. These chapters are tailored to offer practical advice and are further supported by case studies that illustrate the real-world application of mindfulness research in various healthcare settings.
- Embrace Personal Practice: We're going to beat this drum at least a few times throughout the book. For healthcare providers and professionals, it's important to cultivate your own mindfulness practice. This book not only guides you in doing so but also explains why personal practice is key to effectively integrating mindfulness into patient care and healthcare environments.
- Utilize the Resources: Make use of the appendices, which include resources for further reading, mindfulness practice exercises, and guidelines for implementing mindfulness programs or conducting mindfulness research.
- Engage with Technology Mindfully: The chapter on mindfulness and technology offers insights into how digital tools can aid in mindfulness practices while also urging a thoughtful approach to technology use in our personal and professional lives. These chapters are designed for those of us in healthcare to take a step back and take control of the tech around us, understanding what is the new normal and how to incorporate it effectively. Here's the keyword to address the buzz of technology constantly around us, "Bookend." This word and practice, which we will delve upon, should be carried around in your pocket along with your iPhone.

- Reflect and Apply: After each chapter, take a moment to reflect on how the insights and information can be applied in your daily professional practice. And again, take notes, and ideally begin a journaling process if you haven't already. Consistently ask yourself throughout this text, "how does this apply to me, my role in healthcare, and the environment I work in? What actionable items can I bring to work or start at home after having read this text?" Consider discussing key points with colleagues or in training sessions to foster a culture of mindfulness in your workplace.
- Stay Open and Flexible: As you navigate through the book, remain open to the diverse applications of mindfulness in medicine. The field is dynamic, and mindfulness is a practice that can be tailored to various contexts and needs.
- Commit to Continuous Learning: Recognize that the journey into mindfulness is an ongoing process of learning and growth. This book is a starting point, and your continuous exploration and practice will enhance its value.
- Advocate and Share: Lastly, be an advocate for mindfulness in your healthcare community. Share your learnings and experiences from this book with peers, and encourage a collective movement toward a more mindful approach in healthcare.

A concluding chapter will summarize the benefits of a whole-of-profession approach to mindfulness in medicine, and a look at future directions and challenges. Finally, a "call to action" is appropriate, to recognize the gravity of this inflection point in the modern history of medicine and our opportunity to grasp it.

In each of the realms of our ecosystem, from the basic sit-down of a clinic visit to strategic planning for whole health systems, this book intends to be a blueprint for mindfulness in medicine. Let's get started.

References

1. Gunja MZ, Gumas ED, Williams RD II, U.S. Health Care from a Global Perspective. Accelerating spending, Worsening outcomes (Commonwealth Fund, Jan. 2023). 2022.
2. Arias E, Tejada-Vera B, Kochanek KD, Ahmad FB. Provisional life expectancy estimates for 2021. Vital statistics rapid release. Hyattsville, MD: National Center for Health Statistics; 2022.

Chapter 2
Mindfulness 101

Mindfulness has become increasingly popular in mainstream society as a tool for managing stress, anxiety, and depression. However, despite its spreading acceptance, it remains vaguely understood by many, too "squishy," and not concrete enough for others, including many of us in the health sciences.

The popular narratives around the term "mindfulness" itself have shifted away somewhat from the mystical, esoteric, and New Age tropes that have been often associated with it. Mindfulness has roots in Eastern spiritual practices—and also in Western wisdom traditions, including Christian Centering Prayer, Jewish Kabbalah, and Islamic Sufism. Yet it can be conveyed and practiced in a clear, secular way that emphasizes its practical benefits and is accessible to people from all backgrounds and beliefs.

But misconceptions remain. So, what is mindfulness? And what is meditation?

Mindfulness

"Mindfulness" is a broadly defined term that refers to the capacity of the mind to entrain and direct awareness in and of the current moment, in part or in whole. It is the aspect of consciousness that observes our momentary experience.

Jon Kabat-Zinn, one of the pioneers in bringing mindfulness concepts and practices to Western audiences, emphasizes three aspects in his definition [1]: "non-judgmental, moment-to-moment awareness." We can work backward in unpacking it.

- **Awareness:** This capacity of mind is distinct from other aspects of consciousness: sensation, emotion, and thought among them. Rather, it is what attends to and observes these other phenomena of our minds in each moment of experience.
- **Moment-to-moment:** Mindfulness involves our witnessing of the present moment, of our current experience. It is meant to distinguish current observation

from memory (recall of past events, as they may relate to the current state) and speculation (future forecasting). Both are acts of mind separate from the simple, bare experience of the moment. The title of Eckhart Tolle's well-regarded book, *The Power of Now*, nods to this aspect. Mindfulness is our capacity that attends to our "now"—our current experience.

- **Non judgmental:** This aspect is distinguished from reaction and analysis, of our "feeling about" and "thinking about" the observed experience. These phenomena are judgments—generated about the experience at hand, our additional "spin" on the experience attended to. Emotion and thought are capacities of mind different from our mindful awareness, but often inextricably linked with our awareness.

The experience can be framed, at least metaphorically, as a "field" of phenomena in every individual's momentary experience, occurring, ever-changing. Mindfulness is the capacity of our minds that observe that field and its contents. That awareness also includes the broader sense of the field as a whole (in which individual phenomena come and go), and the experience of observing that field (a sense of one's own watching, as it also changes, ebbs, and flows).

It is worth identifying some misconceptions about mindfulness—what mindfulness is not.

- Mindfulness is not a state of "empty" mind, nor an (improbable) attempt to empty our consciousness of any activity or phenomena, nor avoidance of or relief from mental activity. While states of minimal activity may come and go, mindfulness is the basic, intentional observation of whatever state is present. To play off the graphic above, the "snow globe" may be at rest or shaken up into a blizzard; but the observing capacity of mindfulness is simply watching.
- Mindfulness is not an attempt to "force" relaxation. While that outcome often occurs with practice, mindfulness is a state of active awareness, of paying attention to the present moment and its features in consciousness (Fig. 2.1). In this

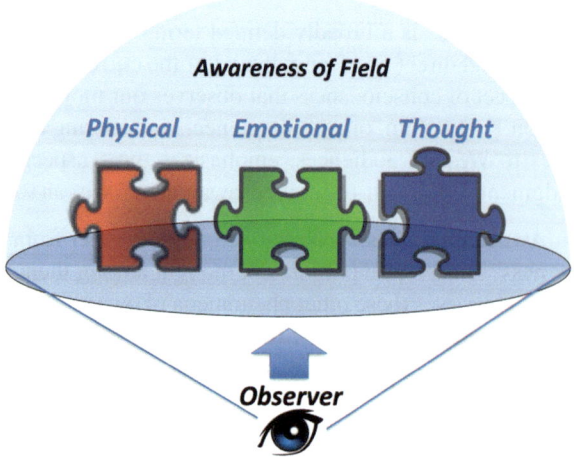

Fig. 2.1 "Field" model of consciousness [2]

sense, it is distinguished from stress management tactics such as relaxation breathing, progressive muscle relaxation (PMR), and guided visual imagery, all meant to induce a state of greater calm and reduced stress. Mindfulness is the capacity of observing consciousness, not intentionally altering the features in observation.
- Mindfulness is sometimes co-mingled with the term "attention," but that can be limiting. Most of us tend to consider attention as directed specifically at a particular, external aspect or phenomenon in our current experience, usually outside of ourselves. Examples would include attention to a child's cry, to a theater performance, or to a question on an exam. Mindfulness certainly involves that but also includes witnessing of "interior" phenomena of the moment, including somatic sensations of breathing, heartbeat and pain, current emotional tone, and thoughts that are being generated. Whether sourced from inside or out, it's all part of the field of mindful observation.
- While, as noted above, cultivating mindfulness has been a feature and goal of many spiritual traditions, it is not a religious practice. Many traditions employ mindfulness practices as a fruitful mode of contemplation. Nevertheless, it is a capacity of a conscious mind that can be practiced by anyone, regardless of their religious or spiritual beliefs.

Mindfulness is a capacity that involves intentional focus of our attention on the present moment, without judgment. It is a capacity that likely predates our intellectual and emotional capacities. Child development specialists presume that an infant's awareness is open, uncluttered, wide-eyed; not yet running self-critical judgments of its state or situation. Of course, that changes as we develop our intellectual and analytic capabilities. But this mindful capacity, while perhaps muted or blanketed by our other aspects of mind, remains available for training and use, all life long.

The broader aim in entraining this capacity is for it to become more familiar and intuitive, to become "built in" as the predominant mode of operating consciously in the day-to-day. In a more attended-to, mindful daily experience, we operate with more deliberation and less reactivity and impulsivity. But that entrainment is less likely without some intentional practice.

Meditation

So, to answer the question, "What is meditation?" we can start there. Meditation is a specific, intentional practice that can help us develop this capacity of mindfulness. Mindfulness is the use of a trainable capacity of mind; meditation is the training, the lesson plan.

Sitting meditation is one type of training practice, well-known and vetted by contemporary research, as we will review later. Yet there are other exercises and practices in cultivating mindfulness, generally focusing on particular physical activities or sensory experiences as the target of observation. These include mindful movement practices such as yoga, Qi Gong, Tai Chi, and walking meditation; mindful sensory observation (music, art, observation of visual/auditory/olfactory detail in nature), and others. One can also practice more informally, observing what is generated in the momentary mind in daily activities such as taking a shower, preparing a meal, or sitting at a stop light.

All meditative practices involve the following:

- There is an **intentional plan of effort in attending to some target or phenomena in current experience** (or many, or all of the "field") in a **purposeful setting and period of time**.
- The plan, simply put, is to, "**attend, lose that attention, and then regain it**"—**limiting additional judgment/thought** in the process and reiteration of that sequence.

Regardless of the type of meditation, the intention of a regular routine of purposeful practice of this capacity is important, as it is for any training, whether running scales on a piano or guitar, employing a foreign language training app, or working on one's putting stroke in golf. That mindfulness is a subjective, "interior" kind of capacity does not change the necessity and benefit of regular, planned practice in developing it.

As for the plan, "simple" may describe the sequence. But the experience of practice is not usually considered routinely simple to do, nor a quick fix. Individuals in meditation variably experience the ebb and flow of sensations, thoughts, and feelings, but also of inevitable losses of attention to reflexive judgments made of the state of the mind at the moment, of excursions into loops of thought about those new entries, and of a dulling out from attention. In the midst of all of these intrusions and distractions from the ideal of a "peaceful, quiet mind," the sequence remains the same: watch, lose the watching, and regain the watching. Try not to get lost in judgment, which is just another form of thinking, while re-engaging the observing intention.

Paradoxically, and important to understand as part of the plan and sequence, is that thinking itself is a double-edged sword to one's development of the focused attention and open awareness that sit at the end of the tunnel. Though the process of thinking is often regarded as the "villainous destroyer" of our meditative strides, it is that thinking itself that allows our mind to ask poignant questions along the way.

After the muddied stages of initial meditative practice are clear and we are better able to sit with our mind and its distractions in a less anxious and fearful way, we may naturally ask some of the most revealing questions of all. We commonly miss these in the initial stages with all its haphazard array of sensations, thoughts, and aimless contemplations.

Instead of making saccadic movements from one distraction to the other, we begin to create space to ask questions as to why we feel or think the way we do in response to any of these sensations, thoughts, or contemplations. Without necessarily spelling it out to us along the way, the mind and its inherent creativity pat down all the natural curves of thought and feeling, uncovering useful pockets of information for long-term contemplation and use, be it during the practice of meditation itself or "off the cushion" in daily life and relationships.

Stated in another way, as we progress through meditation, we allow ourselves to sit with the mind and what may emerge in a way new and different than when we first start.

Setting Conditions

In any form of practice, it is useful to create favored, or even optimal conditions; this is especially true in the most basic form of sitting meditation. In that sense, sitting meditation has these additional factors to consider in that optimization:

- Setting **time** conditions, including a regular schedule (days, time of day) of planning to meditate.
- Setting **space** conditions, involving a setting with minimal additional distracting sensory stimuli—limiting noises and movement in the room or nearby.
- Setting **personal** conditions, including finding one's optimal physical position (traditional meditation cushions, pillow, benches; sitting in a chair, laying down, standing) to be relaxed but alert and attentive. Other factors involve preferences in placement of hands, gaze, and eyes open or shut; all at the discretion of the individual, but with the goal of best aiding the endpoint of cultivating awareness while limiting distraction or discomfort.

A few other factors are useful, not around the concrete tactics of where, when, and how-to, but about attitude in approaching the work. One is commitment to the practice for at least a period of time, regardless of the early struggles or variable return on the investment. Like any training, the initial work can feel too difficult and the benefits are not apparent. Sticking with a regular practice for at least a month or two is reasonable to gain some introductory sense of the benefit on cushion (or chair, or...) and off. But initially, "A for effort""is a good first expectation.

Closely associated with dedication, especially early on, is trying to be patient with the practice and the process. Mindfulness does incrementally develop with practice, in just about everyone. But individual days can be a slog of distraction and tuning out, whether one is a newcomer to meditation or a longtime practitioner. Patience helps (and develops) in both momentary and longer-term senses of the word.

Another attitude deeply treasured in historical guidance on meditation is framed as "beginner's mind," or what the renowned, late meditation master teacher Thich Nhat Hanh [3], referred to as "fresh" eyes. For even an experienced meditator, sitting down with well-worn expectations and pre-conceptions about what is to be experienced can color and limit the meditative practice. "Beginner's mind" refers to the intention to be open to each period of practice, and to each moment in that period, with a fresh sense of curiosity in observation, as we are at the outset of learning to meditate.

Lastly, it's worthwhile to briefly note meditation's own "paradox": that it appears to be an effort to simply be in observation with minimal effort. It can be dissonant to consider a practice where the goal can be seen as no defined outcome, but simply attending to whatever occurs, without a judgment of or action on the experience.

Of course, there is some effort involved—in intention, setting conditions, and specifically in the attending and re-attending of awareness when it is inevitably lost—a conscious effort to simply observe without striving or struggling. The conscious mind is naturally inclined to be active and engaged, constantly moving from one thought or sensation to the next. However, the irony in practice is that the more we try to force our minds to be still, the more active our minds can become. Instead, the key to successful meditation is to approach it with a sense of ease and openness, with a humble, long-term goal of allowing thoughts and sensations to come and go without judgment or resistance (Table 2.1). Creating a comfortable, inquisitive space for the mind to understand what it is experiencing is part of the process of growth. Ultimately, we may appreciate a sensation of discomfort or pain and a thought as the same, the last stronghold of the mind before it relinquishes control to the intense dullness of the experience, repeatedly strengthening one's muscles of attention. Every so often, and likely more common in the later stages of meditation, will be the uncovering of profound personal and objective truths that will allow us to better define ourselves and our relationship with the world around us. Such truths may go hidden for a lifetime if not allowed to be uncovered with this trainable capacity of mindful curiosity.

Learning How

Meditation can be practiced in a variety of ways, with many options available and all valid for an individual to consider, depending on their preferences and needs. The most common, the usual introductory form of meditation, can be called **"focused" or concentrative meditation, which involves directing attention to a specific target in the field or establishing "pointed awareness."** The target can be interior and physical, the breath or heartbeat. Exterior targets can be used, such as gazing on a lit candle or a nature scene. Attending to the felt emotional state of the moment is another interior target. The term "mantra" is well known and often imbued with esoteric or mystical interpretations. In practical usage, mantra simply is a concept, word, or phrase kept in mind (silently or via quiet recitation) as a "thought" object for observation. "Sitting with" ideal states of experience, such as gratitude, joy, or compassion, are yet other concepts that we can observe and attempt to hold in our conscious mind. Regardless of the specific target, we attend to it and watch what develops, noticing when the mind wanders off task and resetting with a minimum of extra judgment, either toward oneself for falling off the horse or toward the experience in general.

Table 2.1 The art and science of meditative practice

Foundational aspects of meditation	• **Intentional effort:** Mindfulness involves purposeful observation of one's current state • **Simple, yet challenging:** The process of attending, losing attention, and regaining it, without judgment
Routine practice importance	• **Regular training:** Like any skill, consistent practice is key to developing mindfulness • **Beyond subjectivity:** Regular practice enhances this "interior" capacity, similar to learning a musical instrument or a language
Dynamics of meditation	• **Ebb and flow of experience:** Recognition of the natural distractions and intrusions during meditation • **Mindful observation:** Consistent focus on observing, losing, and regaining attention • **Thinking as a double-edged sword:** Understanding that thinking can both hinder and aid meditation progress
Deepening understanding through meditation	• **Revealing personal and objective truths:** Meditation uncovers profound insights into oneself and the world • **Mindful curiosity:** Creating space for inquisitive exploration of thoughts and feelings
Optimizing meditation conditions	• **Time and space:** Setting regular schedules and a quiet environment • **Personal comfort:** Finding optimal physical positions and conditions for focused practice • **Maintenance of appropriate posture**
Attitudinal factors in meditation	• **Commitment and patience:** Emphasizing dedication and patience in practice • **Beginner's mind:** Approaching each session with openness and curiosity • **Meditation paradox:** Effort in observing with minimal effort, allowing thoughts to pass without resistance

Another broad type of meditation is "**open" or monitoring meditation, which involves opening the "aperture" to whatever arises, without attending to a specific target**. It's being aware of and observing all thoughts and sensations without reacting to them. This type of practice is usually more advanced, as holding attention on the whole field and its varied and changing phenomena can be challenging. It is common for even more advanced practitioners to include both focused, and open types in a sitting; often starting with basic breath meditation as a kind of "warmup" in the humble routine of attending, losing attention, and regaining; then pivoting after some period of time to "opening out," a more free-form witness of the whole field in the moment, inside and outside.

Training in sitting meditation has until recently been either an individual affair with the help of books and apps or with the use of a meditation teacher, whether live or via recordings, that leads individuals through a meditation practice.

Another more direct form of learning can be found in joining informal or formal meditation groups—individuals meeting together regularly to meditate and often to collaborate on reinforcing practice, sharing tips and difficulties, as well as to offer one another mutual support. A particularly potent, but higher commitment option for some involves attending a meditation retreat. Retreats are scheduled, structured periods of time, typically ranging from a few days to several weeks, during which participants focus on developing and deepening their meditation practice. Retreats may take place in a variety of settings, such as monasteries, retreat centers, or natural environments; virtual retreats have also become available. Retreats are commonly led by experienced meditation teachers. Participants engage in periods of seated and walking meditation, as well as other contemplative practices. The opportunity to withdraw to a setting with optimal conditions, away from the distractions and stresses of everyday life, can help cultivate greater mindfulness, clarity, and insight. Retreats are likely the next steps for practitioners who have worked with introductory meditation practices and gained some familiarity and capability; they are more often rooted in spiritual inquiry (Table 2.2).

Applied/"Hybrid" Mindfulness

As noted above, in a strict sense, the practice of meditation is an exercise in observing experience, rather than palliating stress or inducing calm. Of course, many stress management exercises are "hybrid" efforts to use mindful observation to identify and then work to deliberately and voluntarily relax or calm aspects of physical tension.

- **Mindful breathing exercises** involve identifying felt aspects of inhalation and exhalation, and then consciously regulating the breath to enhance relaxation and focus.
- **Progressive muscle relaxation (PMR)** utilizes a "body scan" routine involving attention to physical sensations in the body in a systematic way, often starting at the feet and moving up through the body.
- **Mindfulness-based stress reduction (MBSR)** [4] is a structured program (developed by Dr. Kabat-Zinn) that teaches both basic meditation and stress

Table 2.2 Exploring the varieties of meditation practices

Focused or concentrative meditation	Open or monitoring meditation
• **Pointed awareness:** Directing attention to a specific target within or outside oneself • **Targets of focus:** Can be internal (e.g., breath, heartbeat) or external (e.g., candle, nature scene) • **Mantra meditation:** Using a word or phrase as a focal point • **Ideal states as focus:** Observing and holding states like gratitude, joy, or compassion in consciousness	• **Whole field awareness:** Being aware of all arising thoughts and sensations without specific focus • **Advanced practice:** Requires more skill to hold attention on varied phenomena • **Combination with focused practice:** Often used in tandem with focused meditation for a balanced approach

reduction techniques over the course of several weeks. MBSR is often taught in a group setting and includes both formal meditation practices and informal mindfulness exercises that can be applied in daily life.

Mindful Movement

Other mindful training programming involves the whole range of mindful movement practices. While these can often be framed as not just secular, but physical exercise-based activities, the core intentions in traditional movement routines are of attention to the experience of the body in motion as the "target," albeit a more complex one than simply the breath or heartbeat.

There are many traditional movement practices, mainly derived from Eastern spiritual traditions. Other more contemporary secular programming will often incorporate meditative aspects to their sequences of aerobic exercise, dance, and/or physical rehabilitation. Popular movement practices include:

- **Yoga** is a mindful movement practice that combines physical postures, breathing techniques, and meditation to cultivate present-moment awareness and reduce mental and physical stress. Through intentional movement and breathwork, yoga encourages practitioners to connect with their body and mind.
- **Qi Gong** is a practice that involves brief sequences of slow and intentional movements, deep breathing, and meditation. These movements are designed to stimulate and attend to the flow of felt energy ("Qi" referring to that experienced energy, "Gong" referring to "gathering") in the body, promoting physical and mental health. Qi Gong movements range from simple and gentle to more complex and dynamic, but all are performed with mindfulness and intention.
- **Tai Chi** is a practice that involves a series of slow and deliberate movements, focused breathing, and mental concentration to promote relaxation and stress reduction. The slow series of movements in Tai Chi, also known as Tai Chi forms, consist of a sequence of flowing and continuous movements performed in a slow and relaxed manner. These movements are designed to promote balance, flexibility, and strength, while also fostering mental focus and concentration. Each movement flows into the next, with an emphasis on fluidity and grace, and of holding mindful attention on the experience of that flowing sequence.

Mindful movement is often preferred for individuals who struggle with sustaining physical stillness due to restlessness or pain. Besides the benefits of physical movement for gentle building of strength and range of motion for extremities, joints, and spine, movement can incorporate focused attention practice, in attending to proper technique in holding a pose or completing a sequence of physical movements. It also offers an opportunity for more "open" attention to whatever arises in consciousness—emotional effects, thoughts that arise, a sense of whole field experience—while proceeding through the sequences. This latter benefit becomes more likely once some familiarity is gained with, say particular poses in yoga practice or sequences of movement in Qi Gong or Tai Chi.

In this way, mindful movement practices offer multiple mindful aspects for cultivation. As with other types of meditation, the core intention is the same—observing some aspect of experience (a breath, a motion, and a sequence of motions), and what may arise in consciousness coincident with that observational target, until that attention is lost. Then an apprehension of "lost," then a prompt return to the intention and target.

Mindful Technology

As with virtually every corner of contemporary life, emergence of technology has revolutionized the way we can practice mindfulness training. With the advent of mobile apps, videos, and podcasts, mindfulness practices are now easily accessible and convenient for anyone with a smartphone or computer. Mindfulness apps offer guided meditations, breathing exercises, and other mindfulness practices that can be done anytime, anywhere, making it easier for individuals to integrate mindfulness into their daily routines. It is a common resource for physicians to refer to patients, especially for an introductory trial.

Videos and podcasts have also become popular tools for mindfulness training, providing a visual and auditory experience that can deepen the practice. Videos offer visual guidance for movements, postures, and breathing techniques in practices like yoga, Qi Gong, and Tai Chi. Podcasts offer guided meditations, discussions on mindfulness topics, and interviews with experts in the field, providing a wealth of resources for those seeking to deepen their practice and knowledge.

While current technology has made mindfulness training much more accessible, it can lack customization. Of course, no technology can compare to or replace the personal guidance of a qualified teacher or practitioner. Nevertheless, startling new advances in artificial intelligence (AI) can offer new, innovative opportunities for the future of mindfulness training, leveraging AI technologies to customize and personalize the training. The AI model offers a future of customized meditation and mindfulness tailored to the unique needs of the patient, healthcare professional, and healthcare system. AI modeling also offers the ability to track progress, produce meaningful metric data, and provide feedback to individuals, serving as the future, more sophisticated supplement to in-person training.

Ultimately, the best way to learn how to meditate is to try out different techniques and find what works best for each of us. Experimenting with different approaches can help find a practice that is sustainable, enjoyable, and effective for individual needs and preferences.

A Mindful Life Practice

As with regular physical exercise, a joy of engaging meditation as a lifelong practice is in perceiving self-improvement or "gains," here in focused attention and access to our native empathy and compassion, as opposed to muscle mass. Practitioners routinely report a softening of rigid attitudes and reactivity; an opening to more contentment in daily life; and a "virtuous cycle" desire to fit more mindfulness practice into the day. Idle moments can become informal opportunities to get in a brief meditation "workout" before a meeting or in the seat before flight takeoff. A morning workplace meditation to ground ourselves and our team can go from a one-off trial to a valued, shared routine. A brief sitting while waiting for friends and family to arrive for dinner can become intuitive, as can another in breaking bread, expressing gratitude for those around us.

Moving from the everyday to some unforeseen and less ideal circumstances, meditation can be a profound tool to adapt to the unease, unfamiliarity, and emotional novelty related to traumatic events. While the abrupt effects of "bad surprises" are a part of anyone's life experiences, professionals in healthcare must be aware of and prepared for radical, traumatic events in our midst to cope with and respond to; such is the nature of the work. Mindfulness practice allows us to harness the simple act of attending to the breath to identify and categorize associated stressors, judgments, and other thoughts, ultimately demystifying them and reducing their further, interior harm. Living with a more clear mind during these uncertain, and at times difficult conditions, we can allow purposeful and intentional contemplation to take place, buffered from the impacts of stress.

Dedicating oneself to practice, especially during difficult times, can generate remarkable growth potential for any human being. A longer-term ability to reduce maladaptive responses to new traumatic events and to process them more deliberately and healthily is perhaps the biggest payoff of mindfulness practice. Like an archer practicing purposefully and incrementally to sharpen her skills, with time and effort, what the archer once may have considered a waste of precious time tends to become a cherished lifelong practice—revealing capabilities and adaptability that can help actualize broader purpose in life.

To best understand and benefit from mindfulness, it is important to approach it in a practical way, from incorporating "formal"/scheduled meditation practice into our daily routines to informally integrating mindful attention into everyday activities. By doing so, mindfulness becomes less of a separate activity and more of a way of daily life. By observing our internal experiences with less judgment, we can relax our grip on negative thought patterns and cultivate a greater sense of peace and contentment. Over time, we cultivate a deeper sense of awareness and presence.

For those of us in the health sciences, subjective attributes such as these are laudable but can raise an eyebrow in terms of evidence-based research to prove and reinforce benefit. Good news: the evidence is indeed powerful and convincing (Tables 2.3 and 2.4).

Table 2.3 Integration in daily life

- Regular practice: Meditation is likened to daily exercise routines, contributing to mental and emotional fitness
- Recognizing gains: As with physical exercise, noticing improvements in focus and compassion can motivate continued practice
- Opportunities for practice: Finding moments in everyday life to engage in mindfulness exercises, like before meetings or during quiet moments

Table 2.4 Meditation in challenging situations

- Coping with stress and emotions: Using meditation to manage stress, unfamiliarity, and emotional turmoil
- Breath as a tool: Employing breath control to navigate and categorize stressors and thoughts
- Resilience and growth: Meditation aids in processing trauma and fosters personal growth, akin to muscle recovery and growth in physical exercise

Key Points

This chapter emphasizes the practical application of mindfulness in daily life and highlights its evidence-based benefits.

Understanding Mindfulness

- Mindfulness is a capacity of the mind that involves nonjudgmental, moment-to-moment awareness of the current moment, observing our experience while aiming to limit our reactions to and judgments of that experience.
- Mindfulness is not about emptying the mind or forcing relaxation; rather, it is an active state of awareness. Mindfulness practices can be used for stress reduction and relaxation, but their core purpose is to observe our experiences separate from reactions and judgments.
- While it is rooted historically in Eastern spiritual traditions, mindfulness is not a religious capacity, but rather a physiological trait, and can be cultivated by individuals regardless of their spiritual beliefs.

Meditation and Mindfulness

- Meditation is a specific practice that serves to develop the capacity of mindfulness. It involves intentional focus on a target or phenomenon in our current experience. It is distinct from stress management techniques like relaxation or breathing exercises.
- Different meditation techniques, such as focused versus open meditation, exist to cultivate different aspects of mindfulness.
- Meditation can be practiced individually, with a teacher, or in group settings, and it can also involve special settings, such as retreats, for deeper practice.

Mindfulness Training

- The cultivation of mindfulness can be done via a variety of valid and accessible training tactics and can become a valuable lifelong practice.

- Mindful movement practices, like yoga, Qi Gong, and Tai Chi, combine physical activity with mindfulness.
- Technology, such as apps, videos, and podcasts, has made mindfulness more accessible, with potential for AI customization in the future.

References

1. Kabat-Zinn J. Wherever you go, there you are: mindfulness meditation in everyday life. Hyperion Books; 1994.
2. Sazima G. Practical mindfulness: a physician's no-nonsense guide to meditation for beginners. Miami, FL: Mango Publishing; 2021.
3. Hạnh N, Thích. The miracle of mindfulness: a manual on meditation. Boston, MA: Beacon Press; 1987.
4. Kabat-Zinn J. Mindfulness-based stress reduction (MBSR). Construct Hum Sci. 2003;8(2):73–107.

Chapter 3
The Science of Mindfulness: Research and Benefits

In recent years, mindfulness has emerged as a key concept in both healthcare and scientific research, offering a wealth of potential benefits for mental and physical well-being. As a topic that bridges ancient spiritual practices and modern neuroscience, mindfulness provides a fascinating opportunity to contemplate the intersection of Eastern and Western perspectives on human experience. In this chapter, we will explore the science of mindfulness, beginning with an examination of the neural mechanisms that underlie mindfulness practices and the role of emotions in the brain. We will then discuss the various health benefits associated with mindfulness and the current state of research in the field.

Far from its roots in ancient wisdom traditions, mindfulness is being described today in the context of science—as an expressed trait, relatable to changes in the brain, and with those changes supported by neurobiological and neuroimaging research [1, 2]. Understanding mindfulness scientifically can be compared to understanding any other physiological capability of the human body. In fact, in examining the components of meditation, we find a series of physiological processes, each with their own unique challenges; the breath, refocusing, and bodily posture, all endured for the length of each moment of practice. While it's not a "muscle" per se (a favored analogy in the mindfulness community), thinking of mindfulness in such physiologic terms can make it more relatable. Concepts such as capacitance, contractility, preload, afterload, use, and disuse are metaphorically relevant to mindfulness—a capacity that we can strengthen with effort. Thinking of it as a physical exercise, which it is in part, meditation practice is to consciousness what regular workouts are to the muscles, bone density, and BMI—albeit without a pricey gym membership.

As with traditional exercise, dedicating to mindfulness practices beyond the rigor of daily life, and during especially difficult times, will lead to more appreciable progress. The converse applies also; challenges we face can impede our mindful capabilities of attention and compassion, leading to deconditioning and further disuse. Our capacity to be present with magnetic-like focus and also be nonjudgmentally empathic is just this aforementioned trait, this "muscle" that we can aim to build through meditation and other mindfulness practices.

Moving on from analogies and allegory, this points us in the direction of looking at the more established science of mindfulness. Like any other human process, mindfulness is a complex and concerted capability, with the many co-occurring components of the mind and body that can be understood at anatomical, physiological, and neurobiochemical levels.

First, here's a bit of historical review.

The Roots of Mindfulness

The capacity of mindfulness and its entrainment via meditation practices have their historical foundations in Hindu and Buddhist spiritual traditions. The roots of mindfulness in Hinduism can be traced back to early Vedic texts [3] and the practice of dhyana or meditation, which forms an essential aspect of the eightfold path in Patanjali's Yoga Sutras. In Buddhism [4], mindfulness is known as sati in Pali or *smriti* in Sanskrit, both of which mean to remember or to be aware. Mindfulness is a core element of the Buddhist Noble Eightfold Path, specifically the practice of right mindfulness, which involves cultivating awareness of the body, feelings, mind, and mental phenomena.

Different types and levels of meditation practice have developed since ranging in the level of intensity and spiritual context. Pathways to spiritual realization have been the aspiration for individuals past and present, often involving many thousands of hours, as the contemplative benefits of mindfulness practice are rarely instantaneous, and consistent practice over time has often been necessary for spiritual aspirants to achieve lasting changes.

The capacity of mindfulness is at its root a neuropsychological one, and one adaptable for use in a variety of secular contemporary settings, including healthcare. The more basic levels of practice are capable of providing immense benefits in physical emotional health and wellbeing, apart from and without the necessity of spiritual seeking. In the West, the modern understanding and application of mindfulness have been significantly influenced by the work of Jon Kabat-Zinn, who developed Mindfulness-Based Stress Reduction (MBSR) in the late 1970s [5]. MBSR is an eight-week program that teaches mindfulness techniques to help participants better manage stress, anxiety, pain, and illness. Kabat-Zinn's work has been pivotal in integrating mindfulness practices into mainstream healthcare and scientific research, laying the foundation for a growing body of evidence supporting the benefits of mindfulness for physical and mental health.

The adaptation of mindfulness practices in Western contexts has resulted in a secularization and re-contextualization of these practices, making them accessible to a broader audience without necessitating adherence to specific religious or spiritual beliefs. This shift has facilitated the investigation of mindfulness through the lens of neuroscience, allowing researchers to study the effects of mindfulness on brain function and structure, as well as its impact on various health outcomes. To better understand the relevance of recent research on mindfulness, a brief review is in order of the neural mechanisms involved in emotional regulation and mindfulness's impact on those mechanisms.

Systems and Networks

Over the past few decades, neurologic research has made a significant shift in moving away from an exclusive focus on individual anatomic brain structures to studying their links in systems and networks [6, 7]. This shift has been driven by advancements in technology, such as functional magnetic resonance imaging (fMRI), which have enabled researchers to map the connections between different brain regions and understand how they work together [8, 9] (Fig. 3.1). By analyzing patterns of brain activity and connectivity, researchers have been able to identify functional networks that underlie cognitive and behavioral processes, such as attention, memory, and emotional regulation. A key advantage of this network-based approach is that it allows for a more nuanced understanding of brain function. Rather than viewing the brain as a collection of discrete regions that perform specific functions, researchers can now examine how different regions work together in concert to produce conscious phenomena, cognition, and behavior. This has led to a more integrative and holistic view of the brain, in which the whole is greater than the sum of its parts. This approach has led to new insights into brain disorders and how they arise from disruptions in network activity, as well as target networks to reinforce through both pharmacological and nonpharmacological interventions, such as mindfulness training.

The Limbic System and Mindfulness

The limbic system is a linked group of structures in the brain that are responsible for emotional activation, motivation, and the somatic/emotional loading or "soundtrack" of event memory. It includes several important structures, such as the amygdala, hippocampus, thalamus, hypothalamus, and cingulate gyrus.

The amygdala, an almond-shaped structure located deep within the brain's medial temporal lobes, plays a pivotal role in emotional processing, particularly in the processing of fear and threat-related stimuli. It is responsible for identifying emotionally significant events and generating emotional responses proportionate to the events and their effect, particularly of threat and novelty. It is linked to and communicates with other brain regions to influence emotional experiences, including:

- The prefrontal cortex (involved in cognitive control and decision making).
- The hippocampus (involved in memory formation and retrieval).

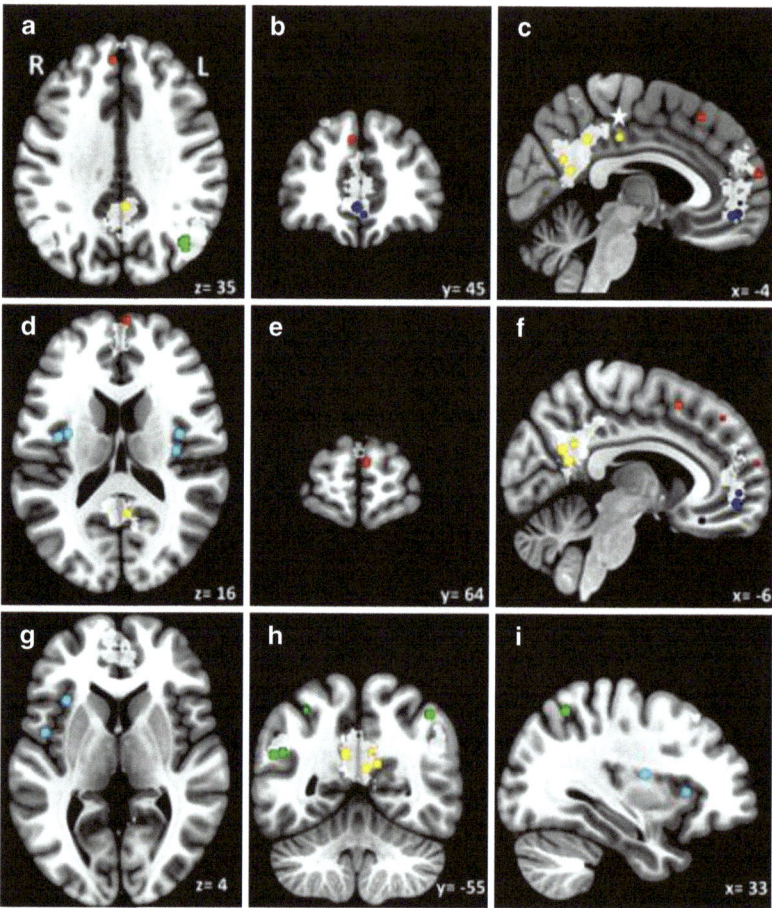

Fig. 3.1 Neural correlates of mindfulness: The involvement of the default mode network and insular cortex in self-related processes and interoceptive awareness

The default mode network (DMN) and the insular cortex play crucial roles in the neuroscience of mindfulness. As illustrated in this figure from Dr. Bruno Weder in "Mindfulness in the Focus of the Neurosciences," self-specifying processes involve the dorsal medial prefrontal cortex (mPFC), while self-relational processes engage the ventral mPFC, pre- and subgenual anterior cingulate cortex (ACC), posterior cingulate cortex (PCC), and retrosplenial cortex. Notably, the involvement of the mPFC at the superior frontal gyrus level is more prominent in individuals without meditation experience, suggesting voluntary effort during task performance. The dorsal area of the PCC, marked by a star, may serve as an interface between the resting state network and the cognitive control network. The insular cortex also plays a significant role, with the proximal insular cortex acting as a primary interoceptive center with distinct homeostatic functions, while the dorsal anterior insular cortex supports explicit interoceptive attention. Furthermore, the posterior part of the inferior parietal lobule (IPL), known as the angular gyrus, is related to the DMN, whereas its anterior part, the supramarginal gyrus, is associated with the frontoparietal control network (FPCN). Understanding the involvement of these brain regions in the context of mindfulness provides valuable insights into the underlying neural mechanisms and can inform the development of targeted interventionsWeder, B. J. (2022). Mindfulness in the focus of the neurosciences—The contribution of neuroimaging to the understanding of mindfulness. In Frontiers in Behavioral Neuroscience (Vol. 16). Frontiers Media SA. https://doi.org/10.3389/fnbeh.2022.928522

- The cingulate gyrus (involved in cognitive processes, such as attention, decision making, and empathy).
- The insula (involved in interoceptive awareness and emotion regulation).

Together, these interconnected brain regions form a complex network responsible for the generation, perception, and regulation of emotions. The network modifies aspects of that emotional processing, including the perception of emotional facial expressions, emotional memory consolidation, and the generation of emotional responses.

Research has shown that mindfulness can have a positive impact on the limbic system [10] (Fig. 3.2). For example, studies have found that mindfulness can reduce activity in the amygdala, which is responsible for the "fight or flight" response [11]. This can lead to decreased levels of stress and anxiety. Mindfulness can also increase activity in the prefrontal cortex, which is involved in decision making and self-regulation. This can lead to improved emotional regulation and impulse control.

By modulating amygdala activity during mindfulness practice, individuals learn to observe their emotions nonjudgmentally and with acceptance, leading to a reduction in reactivity to emotionally evocative events.

As mentioned, mindfulness practices have been shown to strengthen the connections between the amygdala and prefrontal cortex [12]. This enhanced connectivity allows for better top-down regulation of emotions, as the prefrontal cortex exerts greater control over the amygdala's emotional reactivity, allowing more adaptive response to stressors and emotional challenges.

Mindfulness can also have a profound impact on the modulation of intense, hard-to-hold interior states: fear, anxiety, dysphoria, and anger. Becoming overwhelmed or engaging in maladaptive coping mechanisms are common, amplifying, destabilizing secondary reactions to these initial, intense feeling states. These more "primal" coping strategies may quickly dissipate or offload intense tension—but usually generate further suffering and interpersonal difficulties down field. Over time, reinforcement of these maladaptive reactions makes complex and dysfunctional temperaments more likely to occur and persist.

Through the repeated revisiting of these states of mind in the course of regular meditation, adaptation to those initial states is cultivated through better identification of their somatic, emotional, and cognitive components. The formerly hard-to-hold interior states become tolerable, even informative.

Mindfulness, Neuroplasticity, and Neuromodulation

Neuroplasticity refers to the brain's ability to change and adapt in response to experiences, thoughts, and emotions. Mindfulness practices have been associated with neuroplastic changes in various brain regions [13], indicating that these practices can induce lasting alterations in brain structure and function. Recent research has also focused on the modulation of specific brain regions involved in emotion regulation, attention, and pain processing through mindfulness practice. These changes,

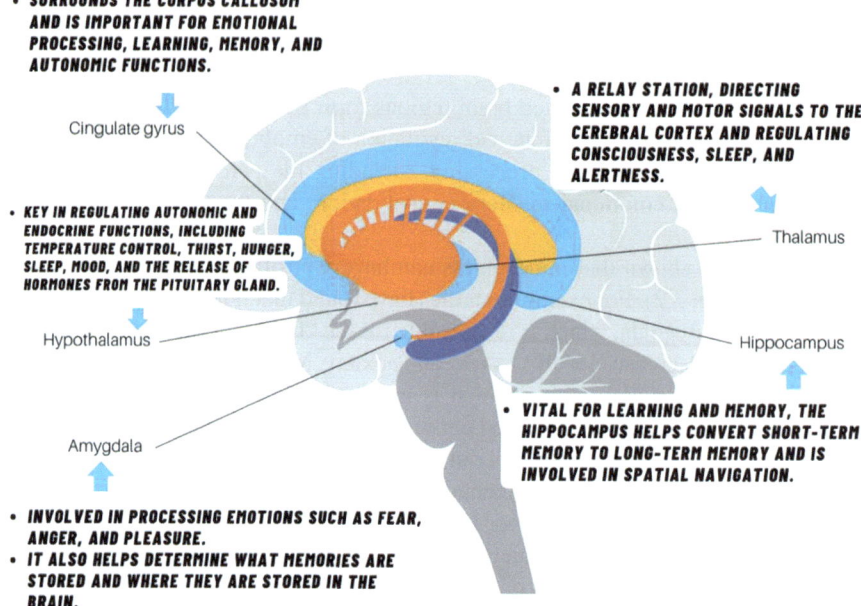

Fig. 3.2 The limbic system and mindfulness The limbic system, an intricate network within the brain, orchestrates emotional regulation, motivation, and the emotive nuances of memories, encompassing structures such as the amygdala, hippocampus, and prefrontal cortex. Central to this network, the amygdala facilitates the processing of fear and emotional stimuli, interfacing with the prefrontal cortex to modulate emotional responses and cognitive appraisal of threats. Mindfulness practice has been empirically demonstrated to attenuate amygdala reactivity, thereby diminishing stress and anxiety responses, while concurrently enhancing prefrontal cortex activity, which is implicated in decision making and emotional regulation. This neuroplastic adaptation fosters improved top-down control of emotional reactivity, enabling more nuanced and adaptive emotional responses to psychological stressors, and refining the management of complex emotional states

seen in neuroimaging research, mirror the functional benefits in reduced suffering and improving emotional wellbeing:

- **Prefrontal Cortex (PFC)**, involved in executive functions and emotion regulation, has been found to increase in thickness and volume following mindfulness practice [14]. This structural change is thought to contribute to enhanced cognitive control and emotional regulation in individuals who practice mindfulness.

- The **hippocampus**, a region involved in learning, memory, and stress regulation, has also been shown to increase in volume [15] following mindfulness practice. This change is believed to enhance memory consolidation, learning, and resilience to stress.
- Studies have reported reductions in **amygdala** volume and activity following mindfulness practice [16], contributing to enhanced emotional regulation and reduced emotional reactivity. As the amygdala is a key region involved in emotional processing and the stress response, these changes are thought to contribute to reduced emotional reactivity and enhanced emotional regulation.
- **Anterior Cingulate Cortex (ACC)** [17], a region involved in cognitive control and emotion regulation, has been found to show increased activity during mindfulness practice. This increased activity is believed to contribute to greater attentional focus and emotional regulation.
- The **insula**, a region involved in interoceptive awareness and pain processing, has been found to show increased activity during mindfulness practice [18]. This increased activity is thought to enhance body awareness and contribute to the modulation of pain perception.

These recent findings on neuroplastic changes and the modulation of specific brain regions are involved in emotion regulation, attention, and pain processing [19]. They provide valuable insights into the neural underpinnings of mindfulness meditation and reinforce our understanding of its beneficial impacts.

Neural Networks and Mindfulness: DMN, SN, and CEN

The linked brain regions that we now identify as comprising the limbic system have been postulated for millennia [20], back to the studies of Aristotle and Galen; and more specifically defined in the 1930s by James Papez as a circuit of brain structures involved in emotion and memory. In the following decades, researchers expanded upon Papez's initial ideas, identifying additional structures and refining the understanding of their functions. Today, the limbic system is recognized as a complex network of interconnected regions that play a key role in regulating emotional and behavioral responses. As research techniques revolutionized neuroscience in the 1990s and forward, three other functional networks have been identified and scrutinized:

The **Default Mode Network (DMN)** is a network of brain regions that is active when an individual is not focused on the outside world, and the mind is wandering or engaged in self-referential thoughts and deactivates during cognitive tasks. The DMN was first identified [21] through studies of brain activity during rest periods. In 2001, researchers discovered a consistent pattern of brain regions that were more active during passive (non-goal-directed-to-task) conditions than during specific tasks, leading to the identification of the DMN. Since then, numerous studies have explored the DMN's role in functions such as self-referential thinking, mental/

imaginal speculation (cognitive "time travel"), and social cognition [22]. This network includes the medial prefrontal cortex, posterior cingulate cortex (PCC), angular gyrus, inferior parietal lobe, lateral temporal cortex, and hippocampus. DMN activity is typically higher during mind-wandering, daydreaming, and rumination—generating secondary mental phenomena, which can be positive, neural, or negative.

In short, the DMN is a kind of "association generator," involved in generating and connecting different types of information, including memories, emotions, and sensory experiences. When the DMN is active, it allows individuals to engage in a variety of mental processes, such as introspection, mind-wandering, and daydreaming, which can be important for creativity and problem-solving. But when the DMN is overactive or hyperconnected, individuals are more likely to generate and reinforce negative, fear-based judgments; they overly worry about the future, or dwell in negative self-talk. In this way, the DMN has been linked to the generation and reinforcement of psychological suffering.

Research suggests that meditation can have a significant impact on the DMN, with experienced meditators showing reduced DMN activity during meditation and increased connectivity between the DMN and other brain networks during rest. This suggests that meditation may help to improve attentional control and emotional regulation by altering the functioning of the DMN and so work to reduce the impact of negative thoughts and emotions. By enhancing attentional control and reducing the influence of the DMN, individuals may be better able to disengage from negative thought patterns and focus on the present moment. Individuals practicing mindfulness experience fewer self-referential thoughts and reduced ruminative thinking, leading to increased present-moment awareness and improved emotional regulation.

The **Salience Network (SN)** was first identified in the early 2000s as a key brain network [23] involved in detecting and filtering "salient" stimuli—information perceived as relevant or significant to the moment and the individual. It's also been found to be involved in other functions and their connections, including attention, emotion processing, and social cognition, allowing for integrating "salient" information with internal states and goals. A prime example: the salience network may be activated when an unexpected or emotionally arousing event occurs, filtering the experience and quickly integrating it with aspects of past experience in memory, and so helping to direct attention and initiate an appropriate response.

It's obvious, then, that the SN is a kind of "relevance alert" system, especially in moments of acute stress. It is directly involved in information management of our cascade of reactions to novelty and threat in the moment. Chronic stress can lead to over-activation of the SN [24], which can result in a variety of negative physical and mental health outcomes, including an increased risk of developing anxiety and depression, as well as physical health problems such as hypertension and cardiovascular disease.

Meditation can also impact the salience network, with experienced meditators exhibiting increased connectivity [25] (Fig. 3.3a and b) between the salience network and other brain regions involved in attention and cognitive control. This suggests that meditation may enhance the brain's ability to detect and respond to salient information in a more flexible and adaptive manner.

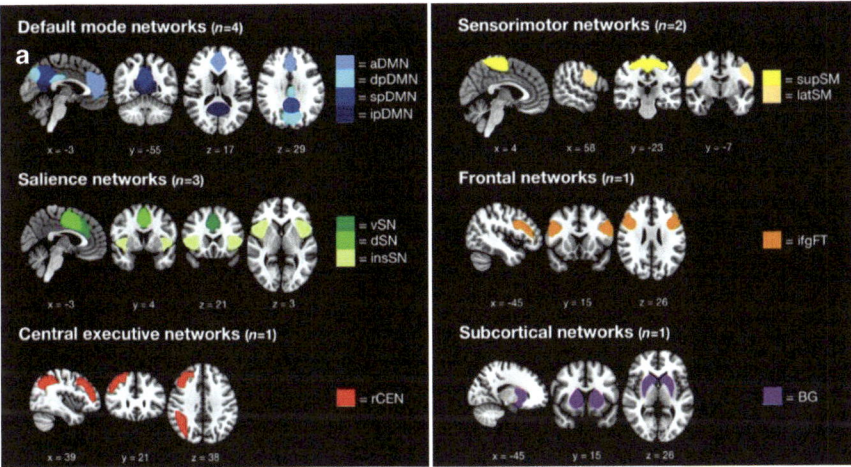

Fig. 3.3 (**a**) Mindfulness meditation has been shown to influence the functioning of large-scale brain networks, particularly the default mode network (DMN), salience network (SN), and central executive network (CEN). Using independent component analysis, researchers have identified 12 subnetworks that can be grouped into these three large-scale networks, as well as sensorimotor, frontal, and subcortical networks. The DMN, which is involved in self-referential processing and mind-wandering, can be further divided into anterior (aDMN) and posterior (dpDMN, spDMN, ipDMN) components. The SN, responsible for detecting and orienting attention toward salient stimuli, includes ventral (vSN), dorsal (dSN), and insular (insSN) subnetworks. The CEN, crucial for executive functions and cognitive control, is represented by a right-lateralized component (rCEN). Additionally, superior (supSM) and lateral (latSM) sensorimotor networks, an inferior frontal gyrus network (ifgFT), and a basal ganglia network (BG) have been identified
Bremer B et al. Mindfulness meditation increases default mode, salience, and central executive network connectivity. Sci Rep. 2022 Aug 2;12(1):13219. https://doi.org/10.1038/s41598-022-17325-6. PMID: 35918449; PMCID: PMC9346127
(**b**) Mindfulness meditation has been found to alter the functional connectivity (FC) between key regions of the default mode network (DMN), salience network (SN), and central executive network (CEN). Using both dynamic FC and seed-based FC analyses, researchers have observed increased connectivity between the superior posterior DMN (spDMN) and two subnetworks of the SN: the insular SN (insSN) and dorsal SN (dSN). Additionally, seed-based FC analysis revealed increased connectivity between the SN and the dorsal posterior cingulate cortex (dPCC), a region functionally associated with the spDMN. These findings suggest that mindfulness meditation enhances the interaction between the DMN, involved in self-referential processing and mind-wandering, and the SN, responsible for detecting and orienting attention toward salient stimuli. Furthermore, the SN exhibited increased FC with regions associated with the CEN, specifically the frontal eye field/dorsolateral prefrontal cortex (FEF/dlPFC) and the supramarginal gyrus (SMG). As the CEN is crucial for executive functions and cognitive control, this increased connectivity may reflect an enhanced ability to regain attention and facilitate cognitive efforts following mindfulness practice-Bremer B et al. Mindfulness meditation increases default mode, salience, and central executive network connectivity. Sci Rep. 2022 Aug 2;12(1):13219. https://doi.org/10.1038/s41598-022-17325-6. PMID: 35918449; PMCID: PMC9346127

Fig. 3.3 (continued)

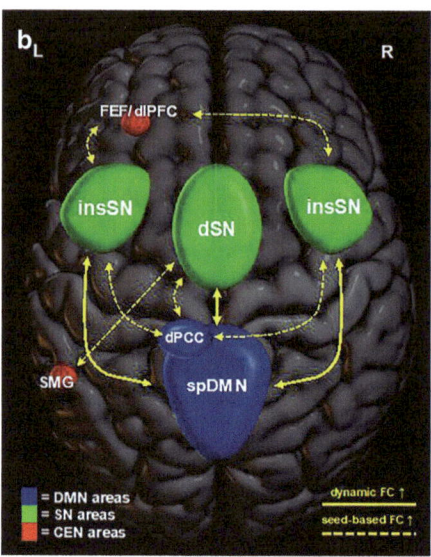

The **Central Executive Network (CEN)** was first described as a neural network [26] involved in executive functions, such as decision making, use of working memory, and cognitive control. The CEN consists of the dorsolateral prefrontal cortex and posterior parietal cortex. It was first identified through functional imaging studies in the 1990s and has since been studied extensively in both healthy and clinical populations. These networks work in tandem to regulate the brain's focus and processing of incoming information. Current research continues to explore the specific roles of different brain regions within the CEN and its interactions with other brain networks.

Meditation can impact the CEN [27], with experienced meditators showing increased activation and connectivity in regions of the CEN involved in attention, working memory, and cognitive control. This suggests that meditation may enhance the brain's ability to sustain attention, regulate emotions, and engage in goal-directed behavior.

These networks work in tandem—generating associative reactions to events, assessing the level of threat and novelty, and framing "executive" responses—to regulate the brain's focus and processing of incoming information and thus allowing individuals to effectively manage our thoughts, emotions, and actions. Mindfulness practices beneficially impact on each of the networks and also change the interaction of the DMN, SN, and CEN. The SN becomes more actively adaptive, helping to focus attention on present-moment experiences and disengage from the self-referential thoughts driven by the DMN. The increased activity in the CEN facilitates cognitive control and the regulation of attention.

This improved dynamic interplay between the DMN, SN, and CEN feeds back virtuously, allowing for further cultivation of mindfulness and improved emotional regulation, changes that are even observable on imaging.

Brain Theory of Meditation

The **Brain Theory of Meditation (BTM)** is an emerging framework [28] that seeks to explain the neural mechanisms underlying different mindfulness practices, including meditation. This theory posits that meditation enhances neural coherence, with implications for consciousness access theories, which seek to understand how information becomes available for conscious awareness and processing. Understanding the BTM can help us further elucidate the neural mechanisms of mindfulness practices, paving the way for more targeted interventions.

- The BTM suggests that meditation practices enhance inter-hemispheric integration, including across the corpus callosum. This integration is known to be central to various cognitive and emotional processes, such as attention, emotion regulation, and decision making. During meditation, increased synchrony between the hemispheres is seen as increased coherence both in electroencephalography (EEG) and functional magnetic resonance imaging (fMRI) studies.
- The BTM also highlights the role of oscillatory coupling patterns [29] in mindfulness practices—patterns of synchronized neural activity across different brain regions. Research has shown that particular and distinct meditation types, including focused/concentrative meditation, open/monitoring meditation, and "aspirational" (gratitude/compassion/loving-kindness) meditation, are associated with their own distinct oscillatory coupling patterns. For example, focused attention meditation is associated with increased gamma-band oscillations, whereas open monitoring meditation is linked to enhanced theta- and alpha-band oscillations. These distinct patterns may be related to the specific cognitive processes engaged during each type of meditation and help explain the unique benefits of each practice.

The BTM is a holistic framework for understanding the neural mechanisms underlying various mindfulness. It has implications for consciousness access theories, which seek to understand how information becomes available for conscious awareness and processing. Mindfulness practices appear to modulate and integrate neural firing, enhancing the brain's ability to improve conscious access to mental phenomena. This enhanced access may promote self-awareness, insight, and self-regulation, which are key components of psychological well-being.

Further research on the BTM and its component processes can contribute to a deeper understanding of meditation's effects on the brain and inform the refinement of more targeted mindfulness interventions. That research should include predictors of long-term success with mindfulness practices, such as individual differences in personality, motivation, or adherence, to inform the development of more targeted and effective interventions.

Attentional Networks and Mindfulness

Another set of neuroanatomic byways is useful to understand our brains' connections function, and how mindfulness practices can beneficially impact that function. Attention was once thought to operate via a single pathway, until researchers discovered that it actually operates via two complementary pathways: the top-down or dorsal pathway, and the bottom-up or ventral pathway. Understanding the role of these pathways is essential for understanding how the brain processes information and directs attention.

Drs. Ian McGilchrist and James Austin are both respected scholars in the field of neuroscience who have contributed greatly to our understanding of these pathways of attention, consciousness, and the impact of mercifulness practices on them. McGilchrist is a British psychiatrist, philosopher, and author whose work has focused on the hemispheric specialization of the brain, arguing that attention operates via two complementary pathways that are associated with the different hemispheres. In his book, *The Master and His Emissary: The Divided Brain and the Making of the Western World* [30], he presents a comprehensive analysis of the hemispheric specialization of the brain and how it relates to attention and consciousness. James Austin, a neurologist and Zen meditator, has studied how meditative practices impact the brain and has written several books on the subject, including *Zen and the Brain* [31, 32]. He has studied how meditative practices impact the brain, and in doing so, he elaborated on a framework that highlights the two complementary attentional pathways and how these pathways relate to the practice of meditation. He argues that meditative practices impact the brain in different ways, depending on which pathway is activated.

The **dorsal attentional pathway**, also referred to as the "top-down" pathway, is responsible for spatial awareness and attention. It operates in the upper part of the brain, from the parietal lobes to the frontal lobes. The top-down pathway generates voluntary, directed attention from an individual's frame of reference and logs "what's" from the observer's perspective—attention to the specific entities that we apprehend and relate to from our individual vantage points. Austin describes this attention as "egocentric" since it is a "self" looking at "not-self" phenomena. This pathway is important for tasks such as directed attention, navigation, visual search, and attentional control.

The **ventral attentional pathway**, also referred to as the "bottom-up" pathway, operates in the lower part of the brain, from the temporal lobe to the parietal lobe. It streams continuously and involuntarily, a background awareness of immersion in the whole "landscape" of consciousness. Austin dubs this one "allocentric," referring to the "perspective of things as themselves," not in reference to the individual self. It allows us to perceive the world as a unified whole, rather than just a collection of separate entities. Bottom-up attention generated via the ventral pathways is our base state of awareness, the effortless, self-free awareness presumed to be present and predominant at birth. As infant development proceeds, dorsal/top-down attention increasingly directs us to specific objects and stimuli in the environment, helping young individuals to develop a sense of self as separate from the external world.

While the ventral and dorsal attentional pathways are separate, they work together to direct attention and focus our awareness. The ventral pathway helps us identify the broader field and its objects and changes in our environment, while the dorsal pathway helps us specifically attend and relate to those objects and changes. Together, these pathways allow us to recognize and navigate our world, and to focus our attention on the most relevant and important information.

As individuals practice mindfulness, they develop an increased capacity to shift their attention away from habitual thought patterns and focus more effectively on present experiences. Meditation can help entrain both attentional paths: top-down attention (entrained more specifically with focus/concentrative meditation practice) to perceive events more clearly, and bottom-up attention (entrained more specifically with "open"/monitoring practice) to embed details in a broader field, beyond the self. By doing so, one can discover a sense of immersion in the present moment, separate from the specifics of "me and it," and instead become more aware of the broader field of experience. In this way, meditative practices can help individuals sharpen their attention and become more aware of the broader reality around us.

Mindfulness and Improved Attention: Evidence

The broad impact of mindfulness practices on attention is to build what can be viewed as a kind of attentional "stamina." As we gradually become better able to sustain attention and awareness in the present moment, the felt state of that mindful awareness becomes more familiar in mind and more welcome as a baseline, steady state of daily experience. Distraction becomes better identified, addressed, and modified, rather than persisted in without awareness or insight.

We can observe these changes anatomically, as structural changes in the brain. Studies have found that mindfulness can increase gray matter density in areas of the brain involved in attention and emotion regulation, such as the prefrontal cortex and anterior cingulate cortex [15]. Other research has focused on the functional benefits of mindfulness training on attention and other aspects of cognition.

Jha et al. [33] investigated the impact of mindfulness training on working memory capacity and affective experience in two military cohorts preparing for deployment. The study found that capacity degraded over time in the military cohort without mindfulness training, while those with practice demonstrated improvements. The study suggested that mindfulness training could potentially serve as a resilience training protocol in various high-stress professions and contexts. Since then, mindfulness training is increasingly being used in the military as a tool to help service members manage stress. In recent years, the US military has implemented multiple mindfulness training programs, including the Mindfulness-Based Mind Fitness Training (MMFT) program and Mindfulness-Based Cognitive Therapy (MBCT).

Kozasa et al. [34] compared brain activity in regular meditators and non-meditators during an fMRI-adapted Stroop World-Colour Task model—a cognitive task used in neuroscience to measure selective attention and cognitive control. Meditators showed less activation increase when processing incongruent stimuli, suggesting better impulse control and attention maintenance. The study concluded that meditation training can enhance brain efficiency in attention and impulse control.

Chiesa et al. [35] offered a systematic review of the broader impact of mindfulness training on cognitive abilities, including attention, memory, and executive functioning. Findings included:

- Short-term benefits: an 8-week meditation program on a short-term intensive retreat improves selective and executive attention in subjects with no prior meditation experience.
- Incremental and longer-term benefits: Long-term practices may lead to further improvements in attentional measures and development of unfocused sustained attention; enhancement in memory, particularly working memory appeared related to the amount of meditation practice.

Malinowski [36] examined neural mechanisms of attentional control in mindfulness meditation. His study highlighted the relationship between mindfulness meditation, sustained attention, and attentional control, finding a positive correlation between self-reported mindfulness and performance on attention tests, with meditators generally performing better than non-meditators.

Lutz et al. [37] explored the neuroscientific aspects of "Focused Attention" meditation and its close relationship with cognitive neuroscience concepts of attention. Long-term practice can lead to reduced activation in attention-regulating neural systems and improved performance in attention tasks. The study highlighted expertise-related changes in attentional processing and brain structures, with expert meditators showing less activation in the amygdala, suggesting reduced emotional reactivity.

Van den Hurk et al. [38] explored attentional processing in the context of mindfulness meditation, examining 20 expert meditators and comparing their performance to 20 age- and gender-matched controls using the Attention Network Test. Findings revealed better orienting and executive attention in the mindfulness meditation group, as well as a reduction in error rates for responses with the same reaction time. These insights highlight the potential for enhancing attentional processing efficiency through extensive mental training in mindfulness meditation.

Research proceeds in refining the understanding of mindfulness practices on cognition, especially attention. The benefits of mindfulness extend far beyond the brain, to overall physical and mental health.

The Impact of Mindfulness on Health

Mindfulness has gained increasing attention in recent years for its potential impact on health and well-being. Research has shown that mindfulness can have a positive impact on a range of health issues, including a direct impact on anxiety and its somatic manifestations, and on pain management. Mindfulness training also has a potent indirect impact on health, improving individual coping with the suffering of both acute and chronic illness, and improving adherence to preventive tactics that are a key aspect of promoting good health and wellbeing. As such, mindfulness-based approaches are sensible to integrate into medical and psychological treatments to promote overall health and quality of life.

A summary of the mechanisms of stress and mindfulness begins with the human response to stress. The physiological stress response, commonly known as the "fight or flight" response, is the body's natural reaction to perceived threats or stressors. This complex response involves the activation of two primary systems: the **hypothalamic-pituitary-adrenal (HPA) axis** and the **autonomic nervous system (ANS)**. These systems work together to mobilize the body's resources and prepare for action in response to acute stressors. However, when this response becomes chronic, it can lead to significant negative health consequences.

- The HPA axis is a major component of the body's stress response system, initiating a cascade of hormonal reactions. The process begins with the release of corticotropin-releasing hormone (CRH) from the hypothalamus, which stimulates the anterior pituitary gland to secrete adrenocorticotropic hormone (ACTH). ACTH then travels through the bloodstream to the adrenal cortex, where it stimulates the production and release of cortisol, a glucocorticoid hormone. Cortisol has wide-ranging effects on the body, including increasing blood sugar levels, suppressing the immune system, and modulating metabolism to provide the body with the necessary energy to cope with stress.
- The ANS, which consists of the sympathetic and parasympathetic nervous systems, also plays a crucial role in the stress response. The sympathetic nervous system (SNS) is responsible for the "fight or flight" response, while the parasympathetic nervous system (PNS) is associated with the "rest and digest" response. During acute stress, the SNS is activated, leading to the release of catecholamines, such as adrenaline (epinephrine) and noradrenaline (norepinephrine), from the adrenal medulla. These hormones cause an increase in heart rate, blood pressure, and respiration rate, as well as a redirection of blood flow away from non-essential organs (e.g., gastrointestinal tract) toward the muscles and brain to prepare the body for action.

While the acute stress response can be adaptive and help individuals navigate potentially dangerous or challenging situations, chronic activation of the HPA axis and ANS can have detrimental effects on the body. Prolonged exposure to cortisol can lead to increased inflammation, as well as disruptions in glucose and lipid metabolism, which may contribute to the development of metabolic syndrome, diabetes, and cardiovascular disease. Chronic stress can also suppress the immune system, increasing vulnerability to infections and impairing the body's ability to mount an effective immune response. Furthermore, elevated cortisol levels have been linked to negative mental health outcomes, including depression and anxiety disorders.

A range of downfield health problems become more likely over time, including an increased risk of cardiovascular disease; digestive disorders, sleep disturbances, anxiety, and depressive disorders; and cognitive decline, including earlier presentation of dementia.

Mindfulness training has been shown to have significant effects on reducing the stress-related hormonal effects that modulate the stress response.

- Cortisol, a primary stress hormone released by the HPA axis, has been a major focus in studies investigating the effects of mindfulness on stress reduction. Research has shown that individuals who practice mindfulness regularly have lower cortisol levels compared to those who do not [39]. This reduction in cortisol is thought to be a result of improved emotion regulation and a decreased reactivity to stressors, allowing the individual to respond to stress more adaptively. Lower cortisol levels have been associated with a wide range of health benefits, such as reduced inflammation, improved immune function, and better mental health outcomes.
- Mindfulness practices have also been found to reduce catecholamine levels [40], such as adrenaline and noradrenaline, which are released by the sympathetic nervous system during the stress response. This reduction in catecholamines leads to a decrease in heart rate, blood pressure, and respiration rate, promoting a relaxation response and counteracting the physiological effects of stress. Additionally, by reducing the activation of the sympathetic nervous system, mindfulness can promote a greater balance between the sympathetic and parasympathetic nervous systems, thereby enhancing overall stress resilience.
- Chronic stress has been linked to increased levels of inflammation in the body, which can contribute to the development of various health conditions. Mindfulness practices have been shown to reduce the production of pro-inflammatory cytokines [41, 42], such as interleukin-6 (IL-6) and tumor necrosis factor-alpha (TNF-alpha), which play a role in the body's inflammatory response. This reduction in inflammatory markers is thought to be related to the downregulation of the HPA axis and the sympathetic nervous system, as well as the enhancement of vagal tone, which has anti-inflammatory effects.
- Mindfulness has also been associated with the modulation of the neuroendocrine system, including the regulation of hormones such as oxytocin [43] and dehydroepiandrosterone sulfate (DHEA-S) [44]. Oxytocin, often referred to as the "love hormone," has been shown to have stress-buffering effects, while DHEA-S is thought to counteract the effects of cortisol and support overall stress resilience. Studies have indicated that regular mindfulness practice can increase levels of both oxytocin and DHEA-S, further contributing to a reduction in stress-related hormones and an enhanced capacity to cope with stress.

Over the past few decades, numerous studies have been conducted to investigate the effectiveness of mindfulness-based interventions in reducing stress and anxiety. These interventions include mindfulness-based stress reduction (MBSR), mindfulness-based cognitive therapy (MBCT), and other similar approaches. The evidence supporting the efficacy of these interventions is substantial and continues to grow.

- **MBSR and MBCT:** MBSR [45], developed by Jon Kabat-Zinn, is an 8-week program that combines mindfulness meditation with elements of cognitive-behavioral therapy to reduce stress and improve mental health. MBCT [46], an adaptation of MBSR, integrates mindfulness practices with cognitive therapy techniques, specifically designed to prevent relapse in individuals with recurrent depression. Both MBSR and MBCT have been extensively researched and found to be effective in reducing stress, anxiety, and depressive symptoms in various populations, including individuals with chronic medical conditions, high levels of workplace stress, and mental health disorders [47, 48].
- **Mindfulness and anxiety disorders**: Several studies have demonstrated the effectiveness of mindfulness-based interventions in treating anxiety disorders, such as generalized anxiety disorder, social anxiety disorder, and panic disorder. A meta-analysis by Hofmann et al. [49] revealed that mindfulness-based interventions significantly reduced anxiety and depressive symptoms across various anxiety disorders, with effect sizes comparable to those of established psychological treatments.
- **Long-term benefits on anxiety:** The positive effects of mindfulness-based interventions on stress and anxiety have been found to persist beyond the duration of the intervention. In a study by Carmody and Baer [50], participants who completed an 8-week MBSR program were assessed at 3-month and 1-year follow-ups. The study found that the improvements in stress and anxiety reduction were maintained at both follow-up points, demonstrating the long-term benefits of mindfulness practice in managing stress and anxiety. Furthermore, regular mindfulness practice has been associated with structural changes [51, 52] in brain areas related to emotional regulation and stress resilience, suggesting that these benefits may be rooted in neuroplastic changes.
- In 2015 PREVENT study [53] by Kuyken et al., a randomized controlled trial examining the long-term effects of MBCT on preventing **relapse in recurrent depression**, though MBCT, combined with support for tapering or discontinuing antidepressant medication, was not superior to maintenance antidepressants over a 24-month period in preventing depressive relapse or recurrence, both MBCT and maintenance antidepressants showed positive outcomes in terms of relapse or recurrence, residual depressive symptoms, and quality of life.
- A systematic review and meta-analysis by Gotink et al. [54] included an analysis of 23 systematic reviews covering 115 unique randomized controlled trials and a total of 8683 participants. The study found that compared to waitlist control and treatment as usual, Mindfulness-Based Stress Reduction (MBSR) and Mindfulness-Based Cognitive Therapy (MBCT) significantly improved depressive symptoms, anxiety, stress, quality of life, and physical functioning. The review highlighted the efficacy of these interventions in the adjunct treatment of various conditions, including cancer, cardiovascular disease, chronic pain, depression, and anxiety disorders, and in prevention for healthy adults and children.

This is a fraction of the substantial evidence supporting the effectiveness of mindfulness-based interventions in reducing stress and anxiety, with long-term benefits persisting beyond the duration of the intervention. These long-term effects may be attributed to continued mindfulness practice and the neuroplastic changes that occur within the brain as a result of regular engagement with mindfulness exercises. By reducing emotional reactivity, enhancing emotional regulation, increasing emotional awareness, and modulating fear and anxiety, mindfulness can contribute to improved mental health outcomes.

Mindfulness has also been increasingly recognized as a promising approach to pain management, with growing evidence suggesting that it can help individuals better cope with chronic pain. Mindfulness-based interventions such as mindfulness meditation and mindfulness-based stress reduction have been found to reduce pain intensity and improve pain-related quality of life.

Mindfulness and Pain

Understanding how mindfulness practices can benefit the suffering of pain experience starts with a summary review of the brain's role in the perception of pain. The experience of pain involves complex processes in the nervous system, from the detection of harmful stimuli to the perception of pain in the brain. Nociception is the initial detection of harmful or potentially harmful stimuli by specialized nerve endings called nociceptors, which can be activated by thermal, mechanical, or chemical stimuli. These nociceptive signals are transmitted from the nociceptors to the spinal cord and then to the brain, where they are processed and integrated.

The spinothalamic pathway is one of the major pain pathways in the nervous system and carries nociceptive signals from the spinal cord to the thalamus, a relay center in the brain that processes and integrates sensory information, including pain signals. From the thalamus, pain signals are transmitted to various brain regions involved in pain perception and processing. These brain regions include the somatosensory cortex, which is responsible for processing the location and intensity of pain; the cingulate cortex and insula, which are involved in the emotional and cognitive aspects of pain perception; and the prefrontal cortex (PFC), with an orchestrating role, in pain modulation.

- The primary and secondary somatosensory cortices are involved in processing the sensory aspects of pain, such as its location, intensity, and duration. These brain regions also allow for the discrimination between different types of pain, such as sharp or dull pain.
- The anterior cingulate cortex (ACC) is associated with the emotional aspects of pain, such as the unpleasantness and suffering. It is involved in attention, motivation, and the regulation of emotional responses to pain. The ACC has been found to be particularly active during experiences of chronic pain, suggesting its involvement in the emotional and affective aspects of pain perception.

- The insular cortex (insula) plays a role in the integration of sensory, emotional, and cognitive aspects of pain. It is associated with interoception, which is the perception of internal bodily sensations, including pain. The insula has been found to be activated during experiences of pain and is involved in processing the emotional and sensory components of pain.
- The prefrontal cortex (PFC), which is involved in higher-order cognitive functions such as decision making, attention, and memory, plays a role in pain modulation through top-down regulation and the assessment of pain-related information. The PFC receives information about pain from various brain regions, including the sensory and emotional aspects of pain, and uses this information to assess the threat level of the pain and generate an appropriate response. One way that the PFC modulates pain is by regulating attentional processes. It can shift attention away from pain-related stimuli, reducing the overall experience of pain. Combined with what we've learned earlier about the PFC, we now understand its modulation via meditation as affecting more than one pathway; regulation of fear corresponding to emotional response communication between the amygdala and the PFC and now, regulation of attentional processes to help reduce the physical and emotional experience of pain [12].

These brain regions involved in the pain response are linked with attentional pathways. The PFC is involved in both the dorsal and ventral attentional pathways, responsible for different aspects of attention and contributing to the regulation of pain processing.

The dorsal attentional pathway plays a role in identifying the location and spatial properties of pain and can direct attention to pain-related cues. The PFC is involved in this pathway and can regulate attention to pain-related stimuli, helping to reduce the overall experience of pain. The ventral attentional pathway, which includes the anterior cingulate cortex (ACC) and the insula, is involved in the detection and processing of salient or emotionally significant stimuli. The ACC is associated with the emotional aspects of pain, while the insula is involved in the integration of sensory and emotional aspects of pain. The PFC is also involved in this pathway and can modulate emotional responses to pain through its regulation of the ACC.

Meditation has been shown to be effective in reducing pain perception, and this may be due in part to its effects on the PFC and attentional pathways [55]. Studies have found that meditation can increase activity in the dorsal attentional pathway, which may enhance attentional control and reduce the impact of pain-related stimuli. Meditation has also been found to increase activity in the ventral attentional pathway, including the ACC, which may lead to improved emotional regulation and reduced suffering from pain.

Besides these direct effects on the neurologic pain response, there are indirect effects of mindfulness training—in coping with the suffering inherent in physical pain. Mindfulness practice can help individuals develop a nonjudgmental and accepting attitude toward pain, which can reduce the emotional impact of pain. By increasing awareness of physical sensations and thoughts related to pain, mindfulness practice can help individuals become more comfortable with the experience of pain and develop a more accepting, less intolerant relationship with it. This attitude of acceptance and nonjudgment can reduce the suffering associated with pain and improve overall quality of life.

Evidence from mindfulness-based interventions for pain relief, including Mindfulness-Based Stress Reduction (MBSR) and Mindfulness-based cognitive therapy (MBCT), have shown both reported benefit and even neuro imaging correlates.

- Numerous studies highlight the effectiveness of Mindfulness-Based Stress Reduction (MBSR) in reducing pain intensity and enhancing pain-related quality of life for individuals with chronic pain conditions, including low back pain and fibromyalgia. A systematic review [56] of MBSR's impact on patients with chronic low back pain indicated significant improvements in subjective pain scores and quality of life compared to control groups. This review, which examined studies published between 2008 and 2018, highlighted the potential of MBSR to complement or even replace pharmacological treatments for chronic pain. A randomized trial [57] highlighted the superiority of MBSR over usual care in enhancing function among patients with fibromyalgia. This study emphasized MBSR's approach to changing how symptoms and stress-related thoughts and feelings are experienced, promoting greater awareness and acceptance. A 2017 systematic review and meta-analysis [58] focusing on MBSR for treating low back pain revealed that MBSR was associated with short-term improvements in pain intensity and physical functioning when compared to usual care. Although these effects were not sustained long-term, the study underlined the need for more long-term randomized controlled trials to better understand MBSR's role in managing low back pain.
- Neuroimaging research by Zeidan et al. [59, 60] has identified alterations in brain activity and connectivity within pain-related regions following MBSR, providing evidence for the underlying neural mechanisms of pain reduction through mindfulness practice. Zeidan's 2011 study demonstrated 57% reduction in unpleasantness and 40% reduction in intensity ratings following nociceptive stimuli in a cohort of individuals following 4 days of meditation training. The study utilized fMRI and arterial-spin labeling to identify associations with reductions and increased activity in the anterior cingulate cortex and anterior insula, as well as thalamic deactivation, proposing a so-called "limbic gating" phenomenon. The study also identified orbitofrontal activation, which is implicated in reframing the contextual evaluation of sensory events.
- Recent research by Zeidan et al. [61], partially funded by the National Center for Complementary and Integrative Health, reveals that the pain relief provided by mindfulness meditation is not dependent on the body's natural opioid activity. This insight is crucial for its application in chronic pain treatment. The study, led by Wake Forest School of Medicine and Cincinnati Children's Hospital Medical Center and published in the *Journal of Neuroscience*, involved 78 healthy adults who underwent either mindfulness meditation or a control activity in response to painful heat stimuli. They also received either naloxone, an opioid activity

blocker, or a placebo saline. The study's design included four groups combining these treatments. Notably, participants practicing meditation reported significantly less pain, regardless of whether they received naloxone or saline, indicating that meditation's pain relief operates independently of opioid neurotransmitter pathways. This finding suggests that combining mindfulness meditation with treatments that activate opioid signaling might be particularly effective in pain management.
- A recent 2021 systematic review and meta-analysis [62] by Pei et al. examining the safety and efficacy of MBCT for the treatment of chronic pain demonstrated short-term reduction in depressed mood and increased mindfulness scores; however, there were no significant between-group (MBCT vs. non-MBCT) differences in pain intensity, pain inferences, and pain acceptance at short- and long-term follow-up. The study calls for larger sample sizes, longer follow-up, and rigorous RCTs.

The benefits of mindfulness are increasingly well-documented. Yet limitations and methodological challenges exist in mindfulness research that can impact the interpretation, generalizability, and applicability of study findings. Addressing these challenges in future research is essential to advance understanding of the most effective components of mindfulness practices and to develop more targeted and effective interventions.

Mindfulness Research: Future Directions

As the scientific understanding of mindfulness and meditation practices continues to expand, several avenues for future research hold promise in deepening our knowledge and refining mindfulness-based interventions. Key areas of interest include these:

- Future research should investigate the role of expertise and effort in meditation practice, as these factors may influence the observed cognitive and emotional benefits. Longitudinal studies comparing novice, intermediate, and expert meditators can provide valuable insights into the specific neural changes that occur with increasing meditation experience. Understanding the relationship between the effort exerted during meditation and its effectiveness can help optimize mindfulness-based interventions, ensuring that individuals receive the greatest benefit from their practice.
- Mindfulness research can also explore potential applications in aging and psychopathology. For instance, meditation may have a protective effect against age-related cognitive decline by promoting neural plasticity and reducing inflammation. Investigating the impact of mindfulness on the aging brain could lead to the development of interventions to maintain cognitive function and well-being in older adults. Furthermore, understanding the neural mechanisms through which mindfulness exerts its effects on psychopathology can inform the develop-

ment of targeted interventions for specific mental health disorders. Examining the potential benefits of mindfulness in these contexts will contribute to a broader understanding of its applications in healthcare.
- To gain a deeper understanding of the brain processes and mechanisms underlying mindfulness, future research should incorporate computational modeling and experimental studies. Computational models can help identify the specific neural circuits and dynamics involved in meditation and generate testable hypotheses for experimental validation. By using advanced neuroimaging techniques, such as magnetoencephalography (MEG) and high-resolution fMRI, researchers can investigate the real-time neural changes associated with different meditation practices. Combining computational modeling with experimental studies can elucidate the complex brain processes underlying mindfulness, providing a more comprehensive understanding of its effects on cognition and emotion.

Future directions in mindfulness research hold significant promise for deepening our understanding of the neural mechanisms and potential applications of meditation. By exploring the impact of expertise and effort, investigating implications for aging and psychopathology, and incorporating computational modeling and experimental studies, researchers can continue to refine mindfulness-based interventions and expand their utility in healthcare and well-being.

Mindfulness: Research Limitations

The above citations and many other studies affirm the role of mindfulness as a non-pharmacologic force multiplier in managing pain syndromes, as has been shown for other pathologies and states of suffering.

Despite the growing body of evidence supporting the benefits of mindfulness, several limitations and methodological challenges exist in the field of mindfulness research [63]. These challenges can impact the interpretation, generalizability, and applicability of study findings, making it essential to address them in future research.

- One significant challenge in mindfulness research is the heterogeneity of mindfulness interventions, which can vary widely in terms of duration, format, content, and instructor expertise. This variability can make it difficult to compare results across studies and determine the specific components responsible for observed benefits. Researchers should strive for greater standardization of mindfulness interventions and clearly describe the specific components, duration, and format of their interventions. This would facilitate comparisons across studies and contribute to a better understanding of the most effective components of mindfulness practices. Many mindfulness studies utilize waitlist control groups or treatment-as-usual control groups, which do not control for non-specific factors, such as social support and expectancy effects. The use of active control groups that match mindfulness interventions in terms of time, attention, and sup-

port can help control for these nonspecific factors and provide more robust evidence of mindfulness-specific effects.
- Another challenge in mindfulness research is subjectivity bias, driven by the reliance on self-report measures, which can be influenced by response biases, social desirability, and other factors. This reliance on subjective self-report measures can limit the accuracy and reliability of study findings. Researchers should strive to incorporate objective measures, such as physiological markers, neuroimaging, and behavioral assessments, to complement self-report measures and provide a more comprehensive understanding of the effects of mindfulness. It is also essential to assess the ecological validity of mindfulness research, as much of the research is conducted in laboratory settings or controlled environments. Including real-world assessments of mindfulness practices and their impact on daily life can provide valuable insights into the generalizability and applicability of study findings.
- Many mindfulness studies involve small sample sizes and homogenous populations, which can limit the generalizability of study findings. Furthermore, research participants are often self-selected, which may introduce biases and limit the applicability of results to broader populations. Researchers should strive to include diverse populations in terms of age, gender, ethnicity, socioeconomic status, and clinical characteristics. This would help to enhance the generalizability of study findings and determine the effectiveness of mindfulness interventions across different populations and contexts. The use of larger sample sizes can also help to improve the statistical power and reliability of study findings, making it possible to detect smaller effects and reduce the likelihood of Type II errors.
- Finally, there is a need for more longitudinal research to examine the long-term effects of mindfulness interventions and the sustainability of observed benefits over time. Including long-term follow-up assessments can help to determine whether the benefits of mindfulness interventions are maintained over time and whether ongoing practice is required to sustain these effects.
- Longitudinal research can also help to identify predictors of long-term success with mindfulness practices, such as individual differences in personality, motivation, or adherence, which can inform the development of more targeted and effective interventions.

The benefits of mindfulness are increasingly well-documented. Yet limitations and methodological challenges exist in mindfulness research that can impact the interpretation, generalizability, and applicability of study findings. Addressing these challenges in future research is essential to advance understanding of the most effective components of mindfulness practices and to develop more targeted and effective interventions.

Aside from reducing suffering, mindfulness' benefits extend far beyond ameliorating illness; it can also be a powerful tool for enhancing overall well-being. Regular mindfulness practice has been shown to improve sleep quality, cognitive clarity, and overall psychological resilience.

Mindfulness and Preventive Healthcare: Cultivating Resilience

"Resilience"is indeed a common term, even an overused one in terms of psychology. But it is often misunderstood or not fully grasped. Psychological resilience refers to an individual's ability to adapt, recover, and thrive in the face of adversity, stress, or traumatic events. It is a dynamic and multifaceted construct that encompasses various cognitive, emotional, and behavioral processes that help individuals effectively manage and cope with challenges.

Resilience is crucial for maintaining mental health and well-being, as it enables individuals to bounce back and recover from negative or challenging experiences, rather than being defeated by them, and continue to function in various aspects of our lives. Moreover, psychological resilience has been associated with lower rates of mental health disorders, greater life satisfaction, and improved physical health.

Resilience is not a fixed trait, but rather a dynamic quality that can be developed and strengthened over time. Several factors contribute to the development and maintenance of psychological resilience.

- One key factor is emotion regulation, which refers to an individual's ability to manage and modulate emotional experiences effectively. Emotion regulation helps individuals cope with stressors and maintain emotional stability, preventing them from becoming overwhelmed by negative emotions. Mindfulness-based practices can enhance emotion regulation by promoting nonjudgmental awareness and acceptance of emotional experiences, reducing emotional reactivity, and fostering adaptive responses to stressors. Of particular benefit is enhancing the capacity for decentering: the ability to observe thoughts and feelings as transient mental events rather than identifying with them. Decentering allows individuals to maintain a balanced perspective on their emotional experiences and respond to stressors more adaptively.
- Cognitive flexibility, another critical factor in resilience, is the ability to adapt one's thinking and perspective in response to changing circumstances or new information. This skill allows individuals to adjust their strategies and behaviors to better cope with challenges and stressors. Mindfulness practices can foster cognitive flexibility by promoting metacognition, which is the awareness and understanding of one's thought processes—in a sense, cultivating observation of one's own conscious experience and process, one's own "mind's eye." Mindfulness practices can facilitate the development of metacognitive awareness, allowing individuals to better recognize and manage unhelpful cognitive patterns that may exacerbate emotional distress.
- Adaptive coping strategies are essential for resilience, as they enable individuals to manage stressors effectively and minimize their negative impact. These strategies can include problem-solving, seeking social support, positive reframing, and acceptance, among others. Mindfulness-based interventions can facilitate the development of adaptive coping strategies by fostering present-moment awareness, enhancing self-compassion, and promoting a nonjudgmental attitude

toward one's experiences. By promoting self-awareness, mindfulness practices can also help individuals recognize when they are engaging in unhelpful or maladaptive coping strategies, allowing them to replace these behaviors with more adaptive responses.

Resilience, then, is the overall beneficial outcome of an orchestrated fine-tuning of mental processes, with their correlates in the neural networks addressed above. Research reflecting the benefits of mindfulness training on resilience is voluminous and compelling; please see back notes for research highlights.

There is an additional, but for our profession fundamental, benefit of mindfulness practice. It can help cultivate and sustain empathy and compassion. These are deeply valuable qualities in and of themselves in individual contentment, as well as in cultivating healthy relationships. They are, of course, core aspects of providing good healthcare.

Mindfulness, Empathy, and Compassion

Empathy and compassion, for both ourselves and others, are essential components of psychological well-being. By cultivating nonjudgmental awareness and acceptance of one's thoughts, emotions, and experiences, mindfulness can help individuals develop a kinder, more compassionate attitude toward themselves and others.

Empathy and compassion obviously also play a particular and crucial role in medical practice, as they are essential for building strong relationships between healthcare providers and our patients. Healthcare providers who demonstrate sustained empathy and compassion toward our patients build all-important trust. That leads to enhanced patient satisfaction, better adherence with treatment plans, and better health outcomes.

Healthcare providers who demonstrate empathy and compassion toward their patients are better off, too. We are less likely to experience burnout, as we are better able to connect with our patients and find meaning and fulfillment in our work. The workplace inevitably benefits, when healthcare providers demonstrate empathy and compassion toward each other, it can create a positive work environment and improve team dynamics.

While empathy and compassion are often conflated, they are really two distinct concepts.

- Empathy is the capacity to mirror and understand the feelings of others— to "stand in the shoes" of another's experience. It is a receptive capacity of individuals in observing and appreciating the state of another—physically, emotionally, and mentally. That received/mirrored experience is its own state in the empathizing individual and is not necessarily easy to hold or work with. An empathic reaction to another's joy is quite different from witnessing pain or harm; as such, the experience of empathy can lead to a compassionate response but also can lead to a need to escape or avoid the intense reaction.

- Compassion, on the other hand, is a response to empathy, usually of the suffering of another. It stems from feeling empathy for someone's suffering and also having a responsive intention to alleviate that suffering. Compassion can be thought of as a positive, active response to the pain of others.
- A potent subset of compassion is "self-compassion," referring to the ability to extend understanding, kindness, and support to oneself, particularly in times of personal difficulty or perceived inadequacy. It is anchored by nonjudgmental awareness, the ability to observe our thoughts and feelings while limiting critical self-judgment or condemnation. This nonjudgmental stance allows individuals to recognize their imperfections and difficulties without succumbing to self-criticism or negative self-evaluations, and in so developing a more compassionate and nurturing "inner voice."

The core components of basic mindfulness—of attending to the experience of the moment more closely and carefully, limiting extraneous discursive thought and judgment, and cultivating adaptation to and acceptance to whatever arises—are central to development of empathy, itself a particular moment of of receiving and holding the felt experience of another. It follows that mindfulness practices make empathic experiences, even intense ones, more familiar and "holdable." That adaptation and tolerance of empathic experience in turn allows for a compassionate response, both to ourselves and others, to flourish and become intuitive. This is a special and targeted benefit of practice for those in the care of others, and of ourselves in a fulfilling yet emotionally challenging profession.

Mindfulness and Acceptance

Roughly corresponding to the long-held trope about the brain's hemispheres, we can frame out two complementary operations: "attentional control" (a "right-brain" phenomenon) and "empathy/acceptance" (a more left-brained construct). While the anatomy of these operations is not that clear-cut (as noted above in the various networks and pathways under study), the two distinct operations appear to have synergistic roles in mindfulness growth through ongoing training practices.

We know that while attentional control practices enhance focus and reduce distraction, acceptance training allows for improved emotional regulation and resilience.58 Acceptance training teaches individuals to engage with present experiences in an open and nonjudgmental manner, a fundamental skill for healthcare professionals. It offers us the opportunity to manage our emotional reactions, not just in moments of acute stress but also (and maybe especially) in tedious or frustrating situations that are commonplace in healthcare settings.

This approach, as highlighted in a study by Rahl et al. [57], demonstrates the critical role of acceptance in reducing mind wandering and enhancing focus. Utilizing an n of 147 healthy young adults and a 6-min "Sustained Attention to Response Task" (SART) measure, Rahl demonstrated that acceptance training was important for reducing mind wandering, such that the attention-monitoring plus acceptance mindfulness training condition had the lowest mind wandering relative to the other conditions, including significantly lower mind wandering than the attention-monitoring only mindfulness training condition.

This study underpins the principle of adaptation through acceptance, be it with the unease of the present moment or a monthly email reminder to attend group meditation sessions.

In Summary: The Science of Mindfulness

Mindfulness practices are of immense value for our patients, colleagues, staff, and ourselves in helping generate and sustain resilience in contemporary life. Improved mindful "stamina," generated through consistent practice, co-generates more deliberation and less anxious reactivity and impulsivity. This shift in consciousness, cultivated via mindfulness training, is truly an attainable opportunity for our patients, our peers in care, and ourselves. The benefits for those who engage in practice are broad and measurable. To summarize:

- A reduction in somatic manifestations of stress that plague so many and are a leading driver of healthcare costs is the first and obvious benefit of mindfulness. Stress-related physical symptoms, such as headaches, muscle tension, and digestive issues, can be debilitating and often lead to chronic suffering and significant increase in outpatient visits. By practicing mindfulness, individuals can learn to better identify and manage the physical sensations associated with stress, reducing their impact on health and productivity.
- Mindful self-awareness routinely cultivates a greater sense of control over not only physical but emotional manifestations of stress. Anxiety, depression, trauma-driven suffering, and substance use disorders are more manageable with the augmentation of medical treatments with meditative practices. Individuals can learn to better identify and manage the thoughts and emotions that contribute to stress and its psychiatric risks. Mindfulness helps regulate emotional responses to stressful situations, managing and reducing negative self-judgment and amplifying positive emotions such as compassion for self and others, contentment, and gratitude.
- Cognitive manifestations of stress include difficulty concentrating, memory problems, and difficulties in executive functioning. Downfield effects of these symptoms, like mental fatigue and burnout, contribute to and amplify a range of mental health disorders. By practicing mindfulness, individuals can learn to identify and manage the thoughts and beliefs that contribute to cognitive stress, receiving them in nonjudgmental awareness. This can lead to improved cognitive function, better decision making, and a greater ability to focus and concentrate.
- Interpersonal manifestations of stress impact our relationships with others. Chronic stress can lead to reactive irritability, a tendency toward conflict in the workplace, home (and medical office), and social isolation. By practicing mindfulness, individuals can learn to identify and manage the thoughts, feelings, and

behaviors that contribute to interpersonal stress. A more compassionate and empathetic approach to their relationships with others can develop, which can lead to better communication and greater understanding. This can improve the quality of interpersonal relationships, leading to a greater sense of connection and community.

In short, mindfulness is a force multiplier for our patients. It cultivates adaptation to physical suffering and improves emotional regulation, cognitive function, and interpersonal flexibility. Research has shown that mindfulness-based interventions can be effective in improving most physical and mental health conditions. Mindfulness practices can promote overall well-being, empathy, compassion, and resilience, equipping individuals with the tools they need to navigate life's challenges more effectively.

Key Points
Mindfulness has gained prominence in healthcare and scientific research, bridging ancient spiritual practices and modern neuroscience. It offers many potential benefits for mental and physical well-being.

Neurological Research
- Mindfulness impacts various neural networks, including the Default Mode Network (DMN), Salience Network (SN), and Central Executive Network (CEN).
- The Brain Theory of Meditation (BTM) suggests that meditation enhances neural coherence, improves conscious access to mental phenomena, and contributes to self-awareness and self-regulation.
- Mindfulness practices can impact the brain's two primary (dorsal and ventral) attentional pathways, enhancing attention and awareness of the present moment.

Research on Brain Functions
- Mindfulness practices improve functioning for multiple aspects of brain function: enhancing attentional "stamina," increasing recognition and management of distractions, and improving working memory capacity, impulse control, and overall attentional processing.
- There is mounting evidence of structural and functional changes in areas of the brain related to attention and emotion regulation that correlate with these clinical observations.

Clinical Research on Mindfulness's Impacts on Physical and Mental Health
- Studies show that mindfulness training promotes overall medical health and well-being: showing a positive impact on various health issues, including anxiety, stress-related hormonal responses, inflammation, and coping with acute and chronic illnesses—leading to better medical and mental health outcomes.
- Research has shown that mindfulness-based interventions, such as MBSR, are effective in reducing pain intensity and improving pain-related quality of life in individuals with chronic pain conditions.
- Mindfulness positively impacts psychological resilience—the ability to adapt and thrive in the face of adversity, stress, or trauma, crucial for well-being.

References

1. Goleman D, Davidson RJ. Altered traits: science reveals how meditation changes your mind, brain, and body. New York, NY: Avery; 2017.
2. Michael Sayers W, et al. The emerging neurobiology of mindfulness and emotion processing. Springer EBooks; 2015. p. 9–22. https://doi.org/10.1007/978-1-4939-2263-5_2. Accessed 3 Jan 2024
3. Sharma H. Meditation: process and effects. Ayu. 2015;36(3):233–7. https://doi.org/10.4103/0974-8520.182756.
4. Wynne A. The origin of Buddhist meditation; 2007. https://doi.org/10.4324/9780203963005.
5. Kabat-Zinn J. Mindfulness-based stress reduction (MBSR). Construct Hum Sci. 2003;8(2):73–107.
6. Tang Y-Y, Hölzel BK, Posner MI. The neuroscience of mindfulness meditation. Nat Rev Neurosci. 2015;16(4):213–25. https://doi.org/10.1038/nrn3916.
7. Brandmeyer T, Delorme A, Wahbeh H. The neuroscience of meditation: classification, phenomenology, correlates, and mechanisms. In: Progress in brain research. Elsevier; 2019. p. 1–29. https://doi.org/10.1016/bs.pbr.2018.10.020.
8. Changde D, Li J, Huang L, He H. Brain encoding and decoding in fMRI with bidirectional deep generative models. Engineering. 2019;5(5):948–53.
9. Weder BJ. Mindfulness in the focus of the neurosciences—the contribution of neuroimaging to the understanding of mindfulness. Front Behav Neurosci. 2022;16:928522. https://doi.org/10.3389/fnbeh.2022.928522.
10. Farb NA, Anderson AK, Segal ZV. The mindful brain and emotion regulation in mood disorders. Can J Psychiatr. 2012;57(2):70–7. https://doi.org/10.1177/070674371205700203. PMID: 22340146; PMCID: PMC3303604
11. Kral TRA, Schuyler BS, Mumford JA, Rosenkranz MA, Lutz A, Davidson RJ. Impact of short- and long-term mindfulness meditation training on amygdala reactivity to emotional stimuli. Neuroimage. 2018;181:301–13. https://doi.org/10.1016/j.neuroimage.2018.07.013. Epub 2018 Jul 7. PMID: 29990584; PMCID: PMC6671286
12. Rathore M, Verma M, Nirwan M, Trivedi S, Pai V. Functional connectivity of prefrontal cortex in various meditation techniques—a mini-review. Int J Yoga. 2022;15(3):187–94. https://doi.org/10.4103/ijoy.ijoy_88_22. Epub 2023 Jan 16. PMID: 36949839; PMCID: PMC10026337
13. Siew S, Yu J. Mindfulness-based randomized controlled trials led to brain structural changes: an anatomical likelihood meta-analysis. Sci Rep. 2023;13:18469. https://doi.org/10.1038/s41598-023-45765-1.
14. Lazar SW, Kerr CE, Wasserman RH, Gray JR, Greve DN, Treadway MT, McGarvey M, Quinn BT, Dusek JA, Benson H, Rauch SL, Moore CI, Fischl B. Meditation experience is associated with increased cortical thickness. Neuroreport. 2005;16(17):1893–7. https://doi.org/10.1097/01.wnr.0000186598.66243.19. PMID: 16272874; PMCID: PMC1361002
15. Hölzel BK, Carmody J, Vangel M, Congleton C, Yerramsetti SM, Gard T, Lazar SW. Mindfulness practice leads to increases in regional brain gray matter density. Psychiatry Res. 2011;191(1):36–43. https://doi.org/10.1016/j.pscychresns.2010.08.006. Epub 2010 Nov 10. PMID: 21071182; PMCID: PMC3004979
16. Taren AA, Gianaros PJ, Greco CM, Lindsay EK, Fairgrieve A, Brown KW, Rosen RK, Ferris JL, Julson E, Marsland AL, Bursley JK, Ramsburg J, Creswell JD. Mindfulness meditation training alters stress-related amygdala resting state functional connectivity: a randomized controlled trial. Soc Cogn Affect Neurosci. 2015;10(12):1758–68. https://doi.org/10.1093/scan/nsv066. Epub 2015 Jun 5. PMID: 26048176; PMCID: PMC4666115
17. Tang Y-Y, Lu Q, Feng H, Tang R, Posner MI. Short-term meditation increases blood flow in anterior cingulate cortex and insula. Front Psychol. 2015;6:212. https://doi.org/10.3389/fpsyg.2015.00212.
18. Haase L, Thom NJ, Shukla A, Davenport PW, Simmons AN, Stanley EA, Paulus MP, Johnson DC. Mindfulness-based training attenuates insula response to an aversive interoceptive chal-

lenge. Soc Cogn Affect Neurosci. 2016;11(1):182–90. https://doi.org/10.1093/scan/nsu042. Epub 2014 Apr 8. PMID: 24714209; PMCID: PMC4692309
19. Zeidan F, Grant JA, Brown CA, McHaffie JG, Coghill RC. Mindfulness meditation-related pain relief: evidence for unique brain mechanisms in the regulation of pain. Neurosci Lett. 2012;520(2):165–73. https://doi.org/10.1016/j.neulet.2012.03.082. Epub 2012 Apr 6. PMID: 22487846; PMCID: PMC3580050
20. Roxo MR, Franceschini PR, Zubaran C, Kleber FD, Sander JW. The limbic system conception and its historical evolution. ScientificWorldJournal. 2011;11:2428–41. https://doi.org/10.1100/2011/157150. Epub 2011 Dec 8. PMID: 22194673; PMCID: PMC3236374
21. Buckner RL. The brain's default network: origins and implications for the study of psychosis. Dialogues Clin Neurosci. 2013;15(3):351–8. https://doi.org/10.31887/DCNS.2013.15.3/rbuckner. PMID: 24174906; PMCID: PMC3811106
22. Carroll J. Imagination, the Brain's default mode network, and imaginative verbal artifacts. In: Carroll J, Clasen M, Jonsson E, editors. Evolutionary perspectives on imaginative culture. Cham: Springer; 2020. https://doi.org/10.1007/978-3-030-46190-4.
23. Schimmelpfennig J, Topczewski J, Zajkowski W, Jankowiak-Siuda K. The role of the salience network in cognitive and affective deficits. Front Hum Neurosci. 2023;17:1133367. https://doi.org/10.3389/fnhum.2023.1133367. PMID: 37020493; PMCID: PMC10067884
24. Na H, et al. The modulation of salience and central executive networks by acute stress in healthy males: an EEG microstates study. Int J Psychophysiol. 2021;169:63–70. ISSN 0167-8760. https://doi.org/10.1016/j.ijpsycho.2021.09.001.
25. Bremer B, et al. Mindfulness meditation increases default mode, salience, and central executive network connectivity. Sci Rep. 2022;12(1):13219. https://doi.org/10.1038/s41598-022-17325-6. PMID: 35918449; PMCID: PMC9346127
26. Menon V. Large-scale brain networks and psychopathology: a unifying triple network model. Trends Cogn Sci. 2011;15(10):483–506. https://doi.org/10.1016/j.tics.2011.08.003. Epub 2011 Sep 9
27. Anselm D, Hölzel Britta K, Boucard Christine C, Wohlschläger Afra M, Christian S. Mindfulness is associated with intrinsic functional connectivity between default mode and salience networks. Front Hum Neurosci. 2015;9:461. https://doi.org/10.3389/fnhum.2015.00461.
28. Raffone A, Marzetti L, Del Gratta C, Perrucci MG, Romani GL, Pizzella V. Toward a brain theory of meditation. Prog Brain Res. 2019;244:207–32. https://doi.org/10.1016/bs.pbr.2018.10.028. Epub 2019 Jan 3
29. Lin Y, Gloe LM, Louis CC, Eckerle WD, Fisher ME, Moser JS. An electrophysiological investigation on the emotion regulatory mechanisms of brief open monitoring meditation in novice non-meditators. Sci Rep. 2020;10(1):14252. https://doi.org/10.1038/s41598-020-71122-7. PMID: 32860004; PMCID: PMC7455688
30. McGilchrist I. The master and his emissary. Yale University Press; 2009. ISBN 978-0-300-14878-7.
31. Austin JH. Zen and the brain: toward an understanding of meditation and consciousness. Boston, MA: MIT Press; 1998. ISBN 0-262-51109-6
32. Austin JH. Meditating selflessly : practical neural zen. Boston, MA: MIT Press; 2013. ISBN 978-0-262-01587-5
33. Jha AP, Stanley EA, Kiyonaga A, Wong L, Gelfand L. Examining the protective effects of mindfulness training on working memory capacity and affective experience. Emotion. 2010;10(1):54–64. https://doi.org/10.1037/a0018438.
34. Kozasa EH, et al. Meditation training increases brain efficiency in an attention task. NeuroImage. 2012;59(1):745–9. www.sciencedirect.com/science/article/pii/S1053811911007531. https://doi.org/10.1016/j.neuroimage.2011.06.088.
35. Chiesa A, Calati R, Serretti A. Does mindfulness training improve cognitive abilities? A systematic review of neuropsychological findings. Clin Psychol Rev. 2011;31(3):449–64. https://doi.org/10.1016/j.cpr.2010.11.003.
36. Malinowski P. Neural mechanisms of attentional control in mindfulness meditation. Front Neurosci. 2013;7:8. https://doi.org/10.3389/fnins.2013.00008.

References

37. Lutz A, Slagter HA, Dunne JD, Davidson RJ. Attention regulation and monitoring in meditation. Trends Cogn Sci. 2008;12(4):163–9. https://doi.org/10.1016/j.tics.2008.01.005.
38. van den Hurk PAM, Giommi F, Gielen SC, Speckens AEM, Barendregt HP. Greater efficiency in attentional processing related to mindfulness meditation. Q J Exp Psychol. 2010;63(6):1168–80. https://doi.org/10.1080/17470210903249365.
39. Turakitwanakan W, Mekseepralard C, Busarakumtragul P. Effects of mindfulness meditation on serum cortisol of medical students. J Med Assoc Thail. 2013;96(Suppl 1):S90–5.
40. Jung Y-H, et al. The effects of mind–body training on stress reduction, positive affect, and plasma catecholamines. Neurosci Lett. 2010;479(2):138–42. https://doi.org/10.1016/j.neulet.2010.05.048.
41. Sanada K, et al. Effects of mindfulness-based interventions on biomarkers in healthy and cancer populations: a systematic review. BMC Complement Altern Med. 2017;17(1):125. https://doi.org/10.1186/s12906-017-1638-y.
42. Walsh E, et al. Brief mindfulness training reduces salivary IL-6 and TNF-α in young women with depressive symptomatology. J Consult Clin Psychol. 2016;84(10):887–97. https://doi.org/10.1037/ccp0000122.
43. Bellosta-Batalla M, et al. Brief mindfulness session improves mood and increases salivary oxytocin in psychology students. Stress Health. 2020;36(4):469–77. https://doi.org/10.1002/smi.2942.
44. Jørgensen MA, et al. Effect of mindfulness-based stress reduction on dehydroepiandrosterone-sulfate in adults with self-reported stress. A randomized trial. Clin Transl Sci. 2021;14(6):2360–9. https://doi.org/10.1111/cts.13100. Accessed 22 Sept. 2021
45. Kabat-Zinn J. Full catastrophe living: using the wisdom of your body and mind to face stress, pain, and illness. Delta Trade Paperbacks; 1991. ISBN 0-385-30312-2.
46. Sipe WEB, Eisendrath SJ. Mindfulness-based cognitive therapy: theory and practice. Can J Psychiatry. 2012;57(2):63–9. https://doi.org/10.1177/070674371205700202. ISSN 1497-0015. PMID 22340145. S2CID 6343661
47. Goyal M, Singh S, Sibinga EM, Gould NF, Rowland-Seymour A, Sharma R, Berger Z, Sleicher D, Maron DD, Shihab HM, Ranasinghe PD, Linn S, Saha S, Bass EB, Haythornthwaite JA. Meditation programs for psychological stress and Well-being: a systematic review and meta-analysis. JAMA Intern Med. 2014;174(3):357–68. https://doi.org/10.1001/jamainternmed.2013.13018. PMID: 24395196; PMCID: PMC4142584
48. Khoury B, Sharma M, Rush SE, Fournier C. Mindfulness-based stress reduction for healthy individuals: a meta-analysis. J Psychosom Res. 2015;78(6):519–28. https://doi.org/10.1016/j.jpsychores.2015.03.009. Epub 2015 Mar 20
49. Hofmann SG, et al. The effect of mindfulness-based therapy on anxiety and depression: a meta-analytic review. J Consult Clin Psychol. 2010;78(2):169–83., www.ncbi.nlm.nih.gov/pmc/articles/PMC2848393/. https://doi.org/10.1037/a0018555.
50. Carmody J, Baer RA. Relationships between mindfulness practice and levels of mindfulness, medical and psychological symptoms and well-being in a mindfulness-based stress reduction program. J Behav Med. 2008;31:23–33.
51. Gotink RA, et al. 8-week mindfulness based stress reduction induces brain changes similar to traditional long-term meditation practice—a systematic review. Brain Cogn. 2016;108:32–41., www.sciencedirect.com/science/article/abs/pii/S0278262616301312. https://doi.org/10.1016/j.bandc.2016.07.001.
52. Marchand WR. Neural mechanisms of mindfulness and meditation: evidence from neuroimaging studies. World J Radiol. 2014;6(7):471. www.ncbi.nlm.nih.gov/pmc/articles/PMC4109098/. https://doi.org/10.4329/wjr.v6.i7.471.
53. Kuyken W, et al. Effectiveness and cost-effectiveness of mindfulness-based cognitive therapy compared with maintenance antidepressant treatment in the prevention of depressive relapse or recurrence (PREVENT): a randomised controlled trial. Lancet. 2015;386(9988):63–73., www.thelancet.com/journals/lancet/article/PIIS0140-6736(14)62222-4/fulltext. https://doi.org/10.1016/s0140-6736(14)62222-4.

54. Gotink RA, et al. Standardised mindfulness-based interventions in healthcare: an overview of systematic reviews and meta-analyses of RCTs. PLoS One. 2015;10(4):e0124344., www.ncbi.nlm.nih.gov/pmc/articles/PMC4400080/. https://doi.org/10.1371/journal.pone.0124344.
55. Nakata H, et al. Meditation reduces pain-related neural activity in the anterior cingulate cortex, insula, secondary somatosensory cortex, and thalamus. Front Psychol. 2014;5:117291. https://doi.org/10.3389/fpsyg.2014.01489.
56. Lindsay EK, David Creswell J. Mechanisms of mindfulness training: monitor and acceptance theory (MAT). Clin Psychol Rev. 2017;51:48–59. https://doi.org/10.1016/j.cpr.2016.10.011.
57. Rahl HA, et al. Brief mindfulness meditation training reduces mind wandering: the critical role of acceptance. Emotion. 2017;17(2):224–30. www.ncbi.nlm.nih.gov/pmc/articles/PMC5329004/. https://doi.org/10.1037/emo0000250.
58. Langen WH, Smith SL. A systematic review of mindfulness practices for improving outcomes in chronic low Back pain. Int J Yoga. 2020;13(3):177. https://doi.org/10.4103/ijoy.ijoy_4_20.
59. Pérez-Aranda A, et al. A randomized controlled efficacy trial of mindfulness-based stress reduction compared with an active control group and usual care for fibromyalgia: the EUDAIMON study. Pain. 2019;160(11):2508–23. pubmed.ncbi.nlm.nih.gov/31356450/. https://doi.org/10.1097/j.pain.0000000000001655.
60. Anheyer D, et al. Mindfulness-based stress reduction for treating low back pain. Ann Intern Med. 2017;166(11):799. https://doi.org/10.7326/m16-1997.
61. Zeidan F, et al. Brain mechanisms supporting the modulation of pain by mindfulness meditation. J Neurosci. 2011;31(14):5540–8. www.ncbi.nlm.nih.gov/pmc/articles/PMC3090218/. https://doi.org/10.1523/jneurosci.5791-10.2011.
62. Pei J-H, et al. Mindfulness-based cognitive therapy for treating chronic pain: a systematic review and meta-analysis. Psychol Health Med. 2020;26(3):333–46. https://doi.org/10.1080/13548506.2020.1849746.
63. Zeidan F, et al. Mindfulness-meditation-based pain relief is not mediated by endogenous opioids. J Neurosci. 2016;36(11):3391–7. https://doi.org/10.1523/jneurosci.4328-15.2016.

Chapter 4
Mindfulness in Clinical Care: Modalities

The overview offered in these pages is rooted in this basic concept: mindfulness, a state of nonjudgmental awareness of our experience in and of the present moment, is a powerful tool for improving both physical and mental health, both for ourselves and our patients. Medical professionals are beginning to acknowledge the trainable capacity of mindfulness, cultivated via meditative practices, as a potent factor in improving our patients' treatment and wellbeing, and our own clinical effectiveness and adaptation in a challenging profession. As research continues to shed light on the benefits of mindfulness, it is becoming clear that it acts uniquely as a health amplifier.

Hopefully, these initial chapters have satisfactorily framed out the "what and why" of mindfulness in medicine:

- A clear definition of **mindfulness as a distinct aspect of consciousness,** separate from other aspects such as sensation, emotion, and intellectual cognition.
- A clear description of **meditation and related mindful practices as training exercises to develop a familiarity with this capacity of mindfulness** and its purpose in the incremental development and cultivation of that capacity.
- A cogent framing out of the **neurobiological "backstory"** of how awareness, whether mindful or less so, operates in the body and mind, via the most recent research elucidating neural systems/networks and their complex connections in anatomic and neurochemical terms.
- A convincing summary of the clinical application of a broad range of mindfulness training programming **in patient care, for benefit at the bedside, in the clinic, and in health management resources.**

As healthcare professionals work to close gaps in our understanding of mindfulness, we find that it has a wide range of applications in the medical field. The research studies offered show that mindfulness-based interventions are effective in treating a variety of physical and mental health conditions. Furthermore, mindfulness has a preventative/adaptive effect on the overall stress response and its manifestations and complications of a variety of specific conditions, such as heart disease, chronic pain, diabetes, and depression.

However, in order to fully utilize this tool, healthcare providers must gain familiarity with the "when, where, and how" we can most effectively apply mindfulness training. In order to effectively incorporate mindfulness training into medical care, individual clinicians can and should be equipped with the skills to teach basic mindfulness practices to our patients.

Understanding the basic similarities, distinctions, and best uses of "applied" mindfulness programming, often offered in online or live education curricula / classes for individuals and groups, can unlock these tools for improved medical outcomes. Additionally, we can become well-versed in the variety of referral resources for patients who may need more specialized training.

Finally, it is important for healthcare providers to be aware of target diagnoses that are particularly amenable to mindfulness-based interventions. For example, mindfulness has been found to be effective in reducing symptoms of post-traumatic stress disorder (PTSD), as well as improving quality of life in cancer patients.

In surveying the options for implementing mindfulness training in our clinical works, there are a couple of obvious ways to cover the topic. One is by the mode of teaching/training, which can include:

- **Direct, in-person** provider teaching, whether by **physicians ourselves** or via clinical staff designated and trained as a **mindfulness consultant and educator.**
- **Formal, structured/sequenced education programming** in basic meditation training, which can be offered at hospital and larger healthcare entities, community settings (community centers, places of worship), educational centers (community colleges/adult learning), and nonprofit community service entities (centers for aging, teen health, domestic violence aid, etc.).
- Other formal, structured training programs with a **specific target audience or condition**, and awash in acronyms (MBSR, MBCT, MBPM, DBT, ACT—more detail on these below).
- **Printed/digital resources** for basic meditation via a variety of well-regarded books on the market on mindfulness and meditation, some with a discretely secular, non-spiritual approach and others leaning in a spiritual direction for those that are particularly drawn to that aspect in lowering the bar to access.
- A plethora of quality **digital audio/podcast and video resources**, easily accessible via Internet (YouTube, podcast platforms).
- Dedicated **smartphone applications** that offer both general and directed sequenced training in meditation, often via a subscription model (most popular currently include *Calm, Headspace, Insight Timer,* and *10% Happier*; more are inevitably on the way, and with deepening functionality and benefit as AI is introduced into this realm).

Another, intersecting mode of classification is by the type of clinical circumstance, covered in the next chapter, which can include:

- **Individual medical office visits**, particularly as part of an overall physical examination/wellness visit.
- **Medical office and hospital diagnostic and treatment procedures** (phlebotomy, MRI/CT, mammogram, pelvic/gynecologic intervention; pre- and post-surgical situations), where pre-emptive and acute care training in mindfulness can be used as a stress-adaptive too.
- **Outpatient psychiatric and psychotherapy care**, weaving mindfulness tactics informally into both the direct interactive counseling work and as a symptoms management and contemplative tool in between visits.
- **Intensive mental care settings**, including inpatient psychiatric hospital units, intensive/partial hospital/day treatment programs, and residential treatment facilities for psychiatric and substance use disorders; clinical settings that can accommodate group/class teaching for both brief and intermittent/sequenced programs.

Interactions, conditions, and clinical settings vary. Yet the basic mindfulness model allows for its implementation in many modes, with a potent role for us in improving care outcomes. As for the basic model, it's a basic educational exercise that all healthcare professionals can gain facility with. Like with our first physical exam, blood gas, or spinal tap, the old directive fits here: *"See one, do one, teach one."*

Learning and Teaching Basic Breath Meditation in the Clinical Setting: First, Ourselves

Basic breath meditation is a conceptually simple (but not necessarily easy to practice) technique that involves focusing on one's breath as the targeted "phenomenon" of our awareness. It's portable; it can be practiced anywhere, and anytime, to help our patients manage anxiety, pain, and other symptoms associated with various health conditions. We can and should teach our patients to take a few minutes each day at a minimum to sit quietly and focus on the breath, regardless of condition or degree of suffering.

From that foundation, additional mindful tactics can be considered, tailored to each patient's individual needs. We can work with patients to identify specific health issues or conditions that may be improved with breath meditation. For example, patients with chronic pain may benefit from learning breath techniques to manage pain and reduce reliance on medication.

But first, we can—and need to—gain the skill set ourselves. The "see one" part of gaining competence in teaching breath meditation is straightforward. There are obvious resources (CME, books, digital media, etc.) for observing others teaching this basic tactic, and following along.

Moreover, the practice of sitting in anyone's own observation of experience is a unique, individual one. The experience of and direct benefit of this simple, powerful practice is easily available to all of us, not just our patients—so there is little practical argument against learning the tactics ourselves. So, optimally, we "do one," in preparation for the opportunity to "teach one."

This is a logical expectation. But for many of us in healthcare, we are temperamentally predisposed to outward action, to "doing." Without too much stereotyping, we are in aggregate a clique that is less likely to be temperamentally drawn to self-observation. Even active observation in the clinical exam is traditionally driven by a heightened sense of external/outward seeking—of communicated symptoms, of presented signs, and of subtle changes in the patient's state from visit to visit. It's more CSI, more "Where's Waldo?" and less interior or inward.

This is an obvious but important point; without some personal attempt at and practice of meditation, we have no valid frame of reference on which to help others as we educate them or guide them toward resources. "Faking it" as an educator without some basic personal experience inevitably exposes a gap in our legitimacy. Understanding the foundational steps of stepping back from immersion to observation, the routine of sitting in intentional observation and the inevitable losses of attention in that sitting, and the empathic guidance with that struggle, allows us to teach and collaborate with some "skin in the game." We benefit in having some peership, if not authority, in conveying the basics of this valuable self-care tactic and tool for observation.

As noted above, we can find basic instructions for breath meditation in and from a myriad of resources. Here's a basic example:

First, we set up some conditions to make our meditation practice easier:

- Find **a quiet spot and a period of time** where we are not likely to be distracted or interrupted.
- **Sit in a well-supported chair, or on a cushion** or pillows on the floor.
- **Eyes? Better slightly open**, resting our gaze gently on a spot on the floor a few feet in front.
- **Mouth? Lips closed**, tongue touching the upper palate or back of front teeth. The jaw is relaxed, and teeth may be touching but not forced shut.
- **Hands should be at rest**, either resting on thighs or loosely folded in the lap.

A note on posture is in order. An optimal holding of any individual's posture in meditation is best considered a work in progress—itself a process of entrainment and adaptation, of finding a favored basic posture, then making adjustments based on the day's bodily experience, aches and pains, etc. Adjustments in our seat, back, shoulders, neck, and face (and its own components—forehead, brow, eyelids, tongue, and jaw) in order to find some optimal posture can become their own distractions. Furthermore, discovering and understanding what is passive, at-rest nonreactivity in different muscle groups and parts of the body is just another valid aspect of meditating. For example, how we physically "handle" silence and stillness is itself part of the practice, another momentary phenomenon contributing to the complexity of meditation. As much as meditation is a practice of a return to attention, it is also a practice of a return to a reasonable (if imperfect) bodily posture—a physical form of attention—that can be as easily dissolved without our noticing as any other distraction.

Decide how long for the practice and set an alarm. (beginners usually start with a few minutes, and work up to 20–30 min over time.)

Start by taking a couple of deep, full belly breaths. Then, let the breathing settle to its normal pattern, without any special effort to change or control it.

- **Place the focus of attention on our breathing,** selecting a spot—nostrils, back of throat, or down near the navel—to focus on. This is often referred to as an "anchor" or "home base' to easily return to when the mind inevitably wanders. As meditators become more experienced and confident in their practice, the anchor will become the breath itself.
- **Feel the sensation** of inhaled then exhaled breath, going in and out. Observe. Just be there and witness it. We can attend to each as "in" and "out," or count the breaths to 10, if that helps to keep attention on our breathing.
- **Mind will inevitably wander off that task…** what to do? When we become aware of having gotten off track, a simple "oh," or "got lost" in mind is sufficient; no further judgment or analysis is necessary.
- **Then return** to our intention, to observing our breathing as it enters and exits our anchor points, and proceed—holding, losing, and calmly regaining attention on the breath, until the practice time is complete.
- **Finish.** At the completion of the timed practice, we can take another deep breath or more to reflect on our state and the experience just completed.

At first, it's common to notice that attention wanders off, time after time. With practice, we improve at recognizing the wandering off into thought or dullness, even as it is happening, and resettling into the intention. We become more able to stay in attention for longer periods of time. But this inevitably fluctuates with the ups and downs of daily life; even experienced meditators can struggle with focus in periods of higher stress.

Again, this instruction is not complex in concept. Its practice, however, generates a "landscape" of interior experience, reaction, attentional loss, and "retrieval" unique to every individual. It is fruitful to become at least basically familiar with our own unique landscape, for our own benefit. It allows an opportunity for us to go on to instruct our patients with some empathy and legitimacy.

Teaching Basic Breath Meditation: A Favored Approach

Our teaching role in medical practice is an obvious aspect of the work, but it is often under-appreciated. We regularly educate patients and parents on treatment compliance, healthy nutrition, and symptom monitoring. The most basic breath meditation training is not really a stretch from teaching relaxation breathing, or even first aid. We can, and should, add this to our "core curriculum," regardless of specialty.

Yet, despite a clear opportunity for benefit, the offer to entrain an activity that invites examination of one's own mind can feel very personal to our patients, just as it can for healthcare professionals. It may even be construed as intrusive or out of bounds. As such, a preferable approach should include a brief, cogent explanation of what mindfulness and meditation are—and are not—as an important prerequisite to any offer for direct education or referral. Then an opportunity can be offered, rather than imposed.

It's best to keep it basic when discussing introductory meditation training in a clinical visit. The "ask" can take cues from our standard motivational interviewing skillset. It starts with an inquiry, a description, and then an offer to engage in some training (or a referral thereof):

I'd like to discuss how mindfulness training could help you. You may have heard about mindfulness and meditation. So, what do you already understand about it?

(Inquire first, as mindfulness has become enough of a cultural norm that "starting from scratch" may be unnecessary or condescending.)

Here's a medical understanding of it. Mindfulness is a specific capacity of our minds. It's the basic awareness of and attention to our experience, right now, in the current moment.

Every moment, our experience includes physical and emotional aspects that come and go, as well as the thoughts we can notice. Our capacity to pay attention to all that, that's mindfulness.

(Another checking for clarity can be helpful here to validate some shared understanding of the definition. Next, we can comment on the purpose and benefit.)

Taking some time every day just to watch all that arises in the body, heart and head, it really helps. Research shows it can help with pain, stress, anxiety, and managing many types of medical problems.

Mindfulness helps us adapt to pain and suffering, so it's a useful way to help yourself in addition to our work.

(Identifying individual conditions and stresses for the patient that could benefit from mindfulness training can be helpful here. Next, addressing the training of mindfulness, via practices such as meditation.)

Mindfulness is actually something we can develop and improve with practice. Meditation is one great way to get better at focusing on what's happening at the moment. That includes our inner experience, and also what's occurring outside and around us.

There are other ways, too, like with mindful movement work. That includes yoga, Tai Chi, and other forms. It's something I can help you get started with in terms of learning and practicing, and for you to work on at home.

Before engaging in any final contracting about learning to meditate, an "attitude check" for the work is important to reinforce from the outset. That attitude is twofold: approaching the practice with curiosity and acceptance, and limiting judgment. This is actually a strongly persuasive factor in how prospective meditators decide, as many individuals who consider or even engage a brief trial of sitting can become quickly frustrated by unreasonable expectations of an easily clear or "empty" mind, and quickly quit over self-judgment of perceived failure and/or outward judgment of "this isn't for me." Here's an example of framing the attitude issue:

There's one really important aspect of meditation: the attitude we bring to it. Meditation goes best with an attitude of curiosity about how our minds work. An attitude of having to "get it right," or of critical judgment about how it's going, is not necessary. Actually, while it's unhelpful, it's completely normal to encounter such a mindset during the initial attempts at meditation.

It's more important to have some humility and even compassion for ourselves when it gets difficult, because that'll absolutely happen sometimes. So we try to let go of the judging, and instead just watch for any judgment if or when it comes up. It's really just another thought to distract us, right?

This initial emphasis on keeping an open mind about opening the mind is usually helpful, even novel and liberating. But it can also be a challenge, especially among strivers who want meditation to be another game to win. It's hard for many of us to shake the competitive conditioning we've grown up with, from sports to grades to promotions. But there can be a kind of relief, a permission to let go of the driving and the striving, and just observe. At best, the attitude framing helps reinforce this practice as play, as exploration, with a dividend of calm and relief. Hopefully, it helps with buy-in to make an effort at nonjudgment a core aspect of the practice.

Then, we can ask (not demand, or shame into):

So... does this sound like something you'd like to try? Got any questions?

Usually, there are questions and misconceptions to anticipate. Here are some common ones:

Most people start by watching their breathing as practice. You can count the breaths if you like, or just observe the air going in and out.

It's absolutely normal to lose track, sooner or later. It happens to everybody, and it's nothing to beat yourself up about. We just notice we've lost track, then go back to watching.

Meditation's completely different from "thinking." It's actually about watching. Watching what happens to some part of our experience, or even all of it.

It's not about stopping our minds from having thoughts. No one can really do that. We can work to reduce how much we add to the story with more distracting thoughts. But having thoughts is not "doing it wrong." That's just how minds are.

Usually you can start with a couple minutes, and then go a little longer as you get the hang of the basic "watch it/lose it/oh/back to watching it" pattern. It'll take some time and practice, but most people really benefit over time when they stick with it. Consider, say, four weeks of effort to see how it can help you.

If some interest is clear, we can offer information on introductory training options, based on the resources at hand, including our own direct teaching that can be scheduled at a separate visit. If there's some time in the current visit (10 min as a minimum, so not generally available for most busy outpatient schedules), we can launch here and now into some brief teaching.

The briefest instruction for a short, shared, guided practice can be helpful to lower the bar:

We can try it right now, if that's ok.
We'll go for a minute or so. I'll meditate with you.

(You can use a smartphone timer, or the clock on the wall.)

Get comfortable but alert, like this.

(Sit up straight with both feet on the floor and hands on your knees, to model the physical position.)

Pick a spot on the floor to train your eyes on, or close them if you want.
Select a place to watch your breath - nose, throat, or belly. Watch yourself breathing in, then breathing out.
At some point, you will lose track of that. When you do, without fuss, go back to watching the in and out of breathing.
I'll let you know when we're halfway done. OK, let's start.

(It's helpful to model a couple of deep breaths; and a brief verbal reminder a few seconds in...)

When you lose track, it's ok—just go back to watching your breath.

(Let a minute, or whatever interval you suggested, elapse. Then, call time, and a quick check.)

"OK, time's up. So, what was that like? Did you notice anything? Feel any different?"

This not only reinforces our interest in the patient's experience but also models a shared aspiration for that individual to notice as well.

It's useful to offer patients a handout (see the **Mindfulness In Medicine** website for resources) that has the directions handy for home use. Also helpful is spending a final moment or two on expectations and next steps. It's also a good idea to mutually "contract" to follow up at a subsequent meeting, or via a scheduled phone or text contact in a couple of weeks. Kick around ideas about a favored place and time for practice. Suggesting some daily practice (a few minutes daily at first, then increasing the time until the next scheduled office visit) creates some accountability, however informally. As some proficiency develops, encouraging our patients to "teach one themselves"—to loved ones, family, and friends, even practice together.

Alternatively, a referral can be made to a local or even in-clinic resource.

The "Designated Sitter": An Office Mindfulness Liaison/Consultant/"Champion"

In our clinical offices, colleague(s) or other staff with interest and training in meditation and other mindful practices can play a crucial role in teaching patients about introductory meditation. By designating and training staff members to lead meditation sessions, patients can benefit from their expertise and support in incorporating mindfulness practices into healthcare and stress management routines.

Identified staff members who have a keen interest in mindfulness or meditation can engage training programs (offered live or online) to develop a deeper understanding of meditation techniques and their therapeutic benefits. Training generally covers the content we've explored so far in *Mindfulness in Medicine*—including introductory concepts, the science behind meditation, different styles of meditation, and effective ways to guide patients through introductory practices. Once designated and trained, ancillary clinical staff can incorporate meditation education into patient visits.

By leveraging the expertise of ancillary clinical staff, medical offices can expand the scope of patient care beyond traditional treatments. Incorporating meditation education into their services not only benefits patients by promoting stress reduction and overall well-being, but it also empowers our colleagues to contribute to patient education and holistic care. This role can also extend to providing training and support of mindfulness practices of our other clinical staff colleagues—modeling mindfulness as a foundational benefit for patients and healthcare professionals alike.

Structured Programming

Most **psychiatric and substance use disorder intensive treatment programs** (partial hospital programs and intensive outpatient programs), as well as residential and inpatient units, have adopted mindfulness training due to its potential benefits in stress management and the opportunity in such settings for group learning. Meditation offers individuals in these settings an effective tool for managing symptoms, reducing general stress, improving emotional regulation, and even targeting specific conditions and symptoms.

The benefits of meditation in psychiatric settings are manifold. Regular practice of meditation can help individuals develop greater self-awareness, cultivate a sense of calm, and enhance their ability to cope with challenging emotions. It can promote relaxation and improve sleep quality, which are especially relevant in psychiatric settings where sleep disturbances are common. Meditation can also foster a sense of connection and support among patients, creating a therapeutic community within the treatment environment.

Many **substances use recovery programs**, whether outpatient or residential, often operate within the foundations of the 12-step model. Substance dependence recovery programs can enrich the effectiveness of the traditional, evidence-based 12-step model by integrating mindfulness training [1] into their approach. The 12-step model, widely used in programs such as Alcoholics Anonymous (AA) and Narcotics Anonymous (NA), offers a framework for individuals to achieve sobriety through mutual support, accountability, and working through the steps. Mindfulness training serves as a valuable complement by introducing practices that foster self-awareness, emotional regulation, and coping skills.

In the 12-step model, individuals attend group meetings, share personal experiences, and receive support from peers who have walked a similar path. Mindfulness training adds an extra dimension to this process by teaching participants to be more fully present in the moment and observe with less judgment and acute distress their cravings, emotions, and thoughts. This heightened self-awareness enables individuals to better understand their triggers, internal conflicts, and underlying emotions that contribute to substance use. Individuals in recovery who cultivate mindfulness practice are more likely to make more deliberate and less impulsive choices. They develop healthier coping mechanisms to prevent relapse, foster resilience, and enhance their ability to navigate challenging situations without resorting to substance use. The synergy between the 12-step model and mindfulness training offers a comprehensive approach that addresses both the social support aspect of recovery and the individual's inner journey toward healing and self-transformation.

Referring patients to meditation training in psychiatric settings is commonly done through a multidisciplinary approach. Mental health professionals, such as psychiatrists, psychologists, or social workers, can assess the suitability and readiness of patients for meditation training. They can educate patients about the potential benefits and address any concerns or misconceptions.

Proper screening and ongoing monitoring of patients' well-being and response to meditation practices is essential. Some patients, whether in acute crisis or with chronic suffering, may find meditation difficult or uncomfortable due to past trauma or other psychological or physical issues. It is crucial for healthcare professionals to provide a safe and supportive environment, offering alternatives, modifications to, or opting out from meditation practices when necessary.

Upon discharge, referrals can be made to qualified **meditation instructors or programs** that specialize in working with individuals with psychiatric conditions. Collaboration between mental health professionals and meditation instructors is crucial to ensure a holistic approach to patient care and to address any specific mental health needs that may arise during the meditation training process.

The incorporation of meditation training in psychiatric intensive and day treatment programs, as well as residential and inpatient units, can offer valuable support to individuals with mental health challenges. By addressing potential risks, ensuring a safe environment, and using a collaborative referral process, healthcare professionals can facilitate the integration of meditation as a complementary therapeutic modality, enhancing the overall treatment experience and promoting long-term well-being for patients.

Mindfulness-Informed Treatment Programs /Modalities

The roots of psychotherapy run back in time for a century. The approach first developed by the psychoanalytic movement has revolutionized the understanding of conscious and unconscious processes of our minds. Once-obscure concepts about the ego, defense mechanisms, and resistances are now part of our mainstream cultural understanding. Yet that foundational analytic approach to psychotherapy has shown its limitations in availability, targets for treatment, and research. It can lack clear guidelines and be less efficient in achieving specific therapeutic goals.

Over the past 50 years, psychotherapy programming has branched off in new directions, informed and complemented by behaviorism research. The goal of more efficient and effective treatment has led to mainstreaming more structured, routinized, and manualized approaches. Various evidence-based therapies, such as **Mindfulness-based Stress Reduction (MBSR), Mindfulness-based Pain Management (MBPM), Cognitive Behavioral Therapy (CBT), Dialectical Behavior Therapy (DBT), and Acceptance and Commitment Therapy (ACT)**, have emerged with structured protocols and manualized interventions.

Mindfulness training often has a significant role in these structured psychotherapy programs. The enhancement of participants' abilities to observe and understand their inner experiences can be particularly valuable in structured therapy programs. Incorporating mindfulness training into these programs offers practical skills for managing distress, improving emotional regulation, and increasing psychological flexibility.

Mastering the details of all the various modalities (and their acronyms) that we may refer our patients to is prodigious, and likely unnecessary. Understanding the core purposes and approaches of the most popular and well-regarded ones allows us to refer with confidence and specificity.

Mindfulness-Based Stress Reduction (MBSR)

MBSR [2] is the most well-known manualized stress management program. It has gained widespread popularity and shown positive results in numerous research studies since its inception in the late 1970s. MBSR is designed to help individuals manage stress, pain, and various psychological and physical conditions through the practice of mindfulness. MBSR combines elements of sitting meditation, body awareness practices, gentle mindful movement (hatha yoga), and education to cultivate present-moment awareness and nonjudgmental acceptance of one's experiences, including states of pain and suffering.

The core emphasis in MBSR is on the **relationship and interconnectedness of our somatic/bodily experiences and our thoughts and feelings** about them. As we inevitably color our momentary experiences with some "spin" of discursive thought and judgment, the reflexive "story" that gets generated impacts the total experience, often with threat-driven additional ideation about fear, grievance, and helplessness. That interconnection runs both ways, with stress-induced negative or fearful judgments generating autonomic reactivity downfield, with the familiar panoply of mind/body suffering: muscle tension, GI disturbance, panic anxiety, and amplified experience of chronic pain.

A key shift in perspective generated via mindfulness practice has a particular benefit in MBSR: in identifying interior phenomena of experience (sensations, emotions, thoughts) as **"events" occurring to each of us, rather than personally "owned" occurrences.** More simply, we can watch "events" unfold more accurately as "those," rather than "mine," recognizing that these events are not solely determined by ourselves, but are also influenced by external factors and circumstances. The personalizing ownership of, say, a bout of back pain or a migraine is a familiar, but errant perspective. This has implications for our self-judgment, whether that be self-compassion or additional self-critique for a difficult event. By understanding such experiences as events, we can broaden our perspective and consider the broader context in which they occur, allowing for a more nuanced understanding of our subjective experience and promoting empathy and understanding toward others' experiences.

Mindful awareness practices help demystify how thoughts and bodily sensations interact in the unique circumstances of each individual. A common aspiration framed by this program is developing a different "relationship" with pain and suffering by reinforcing observation of, deliberation on, and adaptation to these difficult states—rather than reflexive reaction and self-judgment.

The program structure in MBSR is somewhat rigorous—an 8-week program of 2.5-h weekly sessions in a group setting (a class size of 10–16 participants), as well as an additional day-long "day of mindfulness" near the end of the program. Participants are expected to practice at home daily, adhering to media reinforcing the week's curriculum. The small group setting is a potent way to share and support cultivation of what can become a lifelong practice. The program requires a significant time commitment and dedication that can be challenging for some individuals to sustain. Additionally, MBSR is a complement, but not a substitute for professional medical or psychiatric treatment. It may not be universally suitable, being problematic for some individuals in acute psychiatric crises, cognitive limitations, or some physical challenges.

MBSR was developed by Dr. Jon Kabat-Zinn, a psychologist at the University of Massachusetts Medical Center, following on his own explorations of meditation while in college, his study at one of the first meditation centers in the West (the Insight Meditation Society in Barre, MA), and culminating in a pilgrimage to study meditation in India, Burma (now Myanmar), and Thailand. During his travels, he trained under a series of meditation masters, delving into the fundamental concepts and meditative techniques of Buddhist philosophy. That immersive experience cultivated in him a profound understanding of mindfulness and laid the foundation for his subsequent work in developing the MBSR program to translate and integrate the teachings of mindfulness into a secular framework, making them more accessible to a broader audience.

Among a multitude of research showing benefits, a 2004 meta-analysis by Grossman et Al. showed positive results for both psychological and physiological health outcomes for adults who received MBSR. Age-appropriate techniques and language for this therapy have been developed for children and adolescents.

Mindfulness-Based Pain Management (MBPM)

While the MBSR approach can be generalized more broadly to physical and emotional suffering, a more specific curriculum has developed that specifically addresses chronic pain, Mindfulness-based Pain Management (MBPM [3]). This training program, taking into account the dilemma and dynamics of pain, is rooted in a particular concept derived from Buddhist philosophy: distinguishing between:

- **"Primary" suffering, defined as the inevitable, physical and other sensations of human living**; these are unavoidable but often transient, impermanent events.
- **"Secondary" suffering, defined as the additional suffering that arises due to our added reactions**, thoughts, and emotions in response to the primary suffering; which can include fear, anxiety, frustration, helplessness, and grief related to the limitations and impact on one's daily life and activities.

MBPM programs work to help participants better identify and distinguish these components in real time, helping participants accept the aspects of the state that are inevitable, yet also cultivate ways of moderating the secondary, self-inflicted aspects of pain. A particular emphasis in MBPM is on cultivating through meditative practice more positive, alternative states of mind. These qualities, including loving-kindness and compassion, can help generate empathy for ourselves and others, all of us are subject to suffering as ubiquitous to human experience.

MBPM programming is a potent adjunct to chronic pain management programs and practices. Its curriculum is available primarily through an international non-profit organization called Breathworks, founded in 2004 by Vidyamala Burch, a lifelong chronic pain sufferer and meditator, who transformed her own experiences into this beneficial enterprise.

Mindfulness-Based Cognitive Therapy (MBCT)

Mindfulness-based Cognitive Therapy (MBCT) [4] is an evidence-based program that combines elements of Cognitive-Behavioral Therapy (CBT) and MBSR, with the primary target of addressing depression and other mood disorders. The primary purpose of MBCT is to teach participants skills to recognize these thought patterns and prevent them from triggering decompensation into more severe depression or anxiety.

While MBSR emphasizes the mind/body relationship in our holding of somatic suffering, MBCT focuses more specifically on psychological difficulties and especially distortions in thought and emotional phenomena. The different "relationship" emphasized here is with our destructive thoughts and associated emotional states, by reinforcing observation of, deliberation on, and adaptation to them—again, rather than reflexive reaction/judgment.

CBT, a therapeutic approach rooted in the work of Aaron Beck and Albert Ellis in the 1960s and early 1970s, stresses the identification of negative or distorted thought patterns that often become entrenched in our daily experience due to familiarity rather than validity. The cognitive therapy researchers, Zindel Segal, Mark Williams, and John Teasdale collaborated starting in the early 1990s and recognized the opportunity of meditative training to help individuals gain better awareness of thought distortions, allowing the application of the principles of cognitive therapy to address, reduce and resolve them.

Like traditional CBT, there are structured programs that resemble the MBSR model and can be found in hospital, psychiatric, and some clinic settings, as well as in a group therapy education model by individual mental health providers with training. Aside from these, many psychotherapists now well-versed in both the central tenets and techniques of both CBT and MBSR, will often weave them into an individualized, integrative/holistic approach to psychotherapy to best fit the needs of the patient and the circumstances.

Dialectical Behavior Therapy (DBT)

In structured therapy programs like CBT, mindfulness techniques have been integrated to help clients recognize and challenge maladaptive thought patterns and develop healthier cognitive processes. DBT [5, 6] combines mindfulness with additional skills training to address emotional dysregulation and self-destructive behaviors. It has gained a particular validation of benefit in individuals suffering from the chronic tension inherent to personality disorders—especially Borderline Personality Disorder (BPD) and chronic suicidal ideation—and is applicable to other psychological conditions. It stands out as an evidence-based, effective treatment modality for the hard-to-treat BPD; in more general referral terms, DBT provides strategies and training for those individuals with persistent/intermittent intense reactivity and emotionality.

Mindfulness is one component of a suite of skills training in DBT. Distress tolerance skills provide strategies to cope with intense emotions and navigate crises, building on the self-awareness and emotional identification benefits inherent in mindfulness practice. DBT also includes work on tactics in interpersonal effectiveness and emotion regulation familiar with CBT. It incorporates these four modes in a structured and comprehensive treatment framework. It typically includes individual therapy sessions, skills training groups, phone coaching, and therapist consultation meetings.

The "D for dialectical" in DBT can seem like a cryptic term. DBT's developer, Marsha Lineman, embraced the idea of holding and working with opposites, of different perspectives and responses to challenges in life— a reframing of earlier psychoanalytic ideas about managing ambivalent or mixed feelings. For Linehan, who has publicly disclosed her own experiences with emotional dysregulation, self-harm, and borderline personality disorder (BPD), the opposing perspectives include embracing conflicting feelings about a person or situation, and working toward both acceptance and change as inevitable in life. This is especially true in the core "dialectic": of accepting ourselves in our current circumstances while simultaneously intentionally working toward our own change and development. This intention toward flexibility in navigating our lives is more tactical and behavioral than earlier psychoanalytic approaches, yet more awareness-and feeling-based than CBT. Mindfulness practices play a powerful role in improving self-assessment, tolerance, and adaptation to the full range of emotional states.

DBT treatment is available through various mental health settings and providers, including outpatient/community mental health clinics, private practice therapists with certification training in DBT (groups and individuals), and hospital-based intensive programs. When searching for DBT treatment, proper therapist DBT training and experience is obviously important, as well as clarity about the structure, coverage, and any additional resources or support services offered.

Acceptance and Commitment Therapy (ACT)

Acceptance and Commitment Therapy (ACT) [7] is a type of psychotherapy programming that is designed to help individuals achieve greater psychological **flexibility**—defined as the ability to fully engage present experience and the psychological reactions it produces, and to make resulting decisions. The "acceptance and commitment" in ACT refer to another dyad of sorts: an acceptance of the current circumstances vs. a commitment to changing them—in the service of a clear sense of one's own values.

ACT was developed in the early 1980s by Steven C. Hayes, a psychologist and researcher. Inspired by his own struggles with anxiety and depression, Hayes sought to create a therapy approach that focused on accepting one's thoughts and emotions while committing to actions aligned with a more conscious definition of and living by one's own personal value set. Research has shown promising effects of ACT with a variety of psychological and physiological health problems such as anxiety disorders, depression, distress associated with psychotic symptoms, chronic pain, epilepsy, trichotillomania, chronic skin picking, and diabetes.

Of ACT's six foundational principles, the first four are mindfulness-based:

- An intention to be in **contact** with present moment.
- **Acceptance** of the current experience (a nod against avoidance and/or judgment).

- Cognitive "**defusion**" (a term for uncoupling from and identifying thoughts as separate).
- **Perspective** taking (a reframing of the observing self as valid and separate from momentary events and reactions).

The last two principles distinguish ACT in terms of the utility of mindfulness toward decision making and action:

- Identifying, clarifying and involving one's own **values** to inform options in the moment.
- **Commitment to action** in the service of one's values, informed by clear understanding of both current experience and the foundation of that value set.

The approach is based on the familiar premise that it is natural for individuals to experience difficult thoughts and emotions, and that attempting to eliminate or control these experiences can be counterproductive. Instead, ACT teaches individuals to accept these experiences and focus on living a values-driven life. The process of values clarification involves identifying the things that are most important to an individual, such as relationships, personal growth, and/or career aspirations. These values are used to guide the individual's actions and behaviors, helping them to live a more meaningful and purposeful life. As with other therapies, mindfulness is used in ACT to help individuals observe and accept their thoughts and emotions, rather than trying to suppress or control them.

Mindfulness-Informed Treatment Programs /Modalities: Which One to Refer to?

While all of the above programs and modalities have aspects of mindfulness training and concepts "baked in," their target conditions and aspirations can differ. As a core training in managing stress, MBSR is valuable as the most evidence-based effective introduction. Specific physical conditions (such as pain) and psychological ones (such as depression and anxiety) have driven their own niche programs.

DBT and ACT are "applied mindfulness" programs that share certain elements; their conceptual differences lie in their primary focus and the strategies employed. DBT places a strong emphasis on developing skills to manage intense emotions and self-destructive behaviors and helps individuals with emotionally complex or painful moments and interactions. ACT, on the other hand, emphasizes the acceptance of inner experiences and values-driven action, utilizing mindfulness training to help individuals toward deliberation in decision making, including committed action toward their values and goals.

Overall, the development of these structured, routinized, and manualized psychotherapy programs in the past four decades has been a response to the limitations of open-ended therapy. The integration of mindfulness training within these programs has proven to be beneficial, as it equips individuals with practical skills to manage psychological difficulties and enhance overall well-being. By combining structure, evidence-based techniques, and mindfulness, these programs offer patients a roadmap for change and empower them to actively participate in their treatment.

Resources for Mindfulness Training

Individuals interested in building the capacity of mindfulness via meditation and other mindfulness practices also have a wealth of print, audio, and digital resources at their disposal. These resources offer valuable guidance, techniques, and insights, enabling individuals to cultivate mindfulness, reduce stress, and participate in their overall well-being. The availability of print and digital resources has greatly facilitated the accessibility and widespread adoption of meditation.

Print resources include books, magazines, and printed guides that provide comprehensive information on various meditation techniques, principles, and philosophies. These resources often offer step-by-step instructions, meditation scripts, and insights from experienced practitioners. The print format allows individuals to delve into the content at their own pace, making it an ideal choice for those who prefer a tangible and immersive reading experience.

Books can run the spectrum from a more spiritual and/or contemplative angle (Thich That Hanh's *The Miracle of Mindfulness*, Eckhart Tolle's *The Power of Now*) to more secular, practical, and clinical approaches (Jon Kabat-Zinn's *Full Catastrophe Living*, Dan Harris' *10% Happier,* Greg Sazima MD's *Practical Mindfulness,* Ronald Epstein MD's *Attending.)* Introductory books provide step-by-step instructions on various meditation techniques and offer insights into the benefits of mindfulness. More advanced practitioners can explore in-depth texts on specific meditation traditions.

Digital resources have become increasingly popular in recent years and offer a convenient and accessible way to learn and practice meditation. Online platforms, channels, and websites provide a wide range of guided meditation sessions, instructional videos, and interactive courses. Websites like Mindful.org and Tricycle.org provide articles, videos, and podcasts that cover a wide range of meditation-related topics. Digital formats provide the advantage of convenience and accessibility, allowing users to access content anytime, anywhere, from their computers or mobile devices.

Podcasts have also emerged as a popular medium for learning about meditation. Numerous podcasts feature interviews with meditation experts, discussions on different meditation techniques, and guided meditation sessions.

Apps like Headspace, The Mindfulness App, Calm, and Insight Timer offer extensive libraries of meditation content, including guided meditations, sleep aids, and mindfulness exercises. These digital resources often cater to specific needs, such as stress reduction, sleep improvement, or focus enhancement.

Online communities and forums provide spaces for individuals to connect with like-minded practitioners, ask questions, and share experiences. These platforms allow individuals to learn from a diverse range of perspectives and gain valuable insights into their meditation practice. Many of these digital resources also offer community features, allowing users to connect with other practitioners, join group challenges, and share their progress and experiences.

Formal, structured/sequenced education programming in basic meditation training, which can be offered at hospital and larger healthcare entities, community settings (community centers, places of worship), educational centers (community colleges/adult learning), and nonprofit community service entities (centers for aging, teen health, domestic violence aid, etc.).

In Summary: A Wealth of Mindful Tools

Mindfulness has a wide range of applications for us in healthcare, supported by research showing its effectiveness in treating physical and mental health conditions and a preventative/adaptive effect on the overall stress response. But as a profession, to fully utilize mindfulness as a tool, we need to understand them better to use and recommend them—when, where, and how to apply mindfulness training effectively. We can master the skills to teach basic mindfulness practices to patients. We can and should become familiar with the main live, published, and digital education curricula for both basic and "applied" mindfulness programming and the referral resources thereof. For diagnoses that are particularly receptive to mindfulness-based interventions, such as chronic pain, depression, PTSD, and cancer, providing patients with this additional tool for improving their well-being should become an essential part of treatment planning.

It is also important for us to identify and target the specific situations and settings where mindfulness practices can help in the moment. That review is next.

Key Points

Mindfulness in Clinical Care Settings
- Mindfulness has proven to be a powerful tool for improving both physical and mental health in both patients and healthcare professionals.
- Healthcare providers must become familiar with the "when, where, and how" of applying mindfulness training in clinical care, equipping themselves to teach basic mindfulness practices to patients and referring those in need of specialized training.

Learning and Teaching Basic Breath Meditation in the Clinical Setting
- Basic breath meditation involves focusing on one's breath as a means to manage anxiety, pain, and other symptoms associated with health conditions.

- Healthcare professionals should first gain the skill set themselves through observation and practice, understanding that personal experience is crucial in teaching and guiding patients effectively.
- Teaching breath meditation involves creating a favorable environment for patients to explore mindfulness, emphasizing an attitude of curiosity and acceptance, and offering brief, cogent explanations and guided practices.

Teaching Basic Breath Meditation
- Healthcare professionals can introduce mindfulness to patients by starting with an inquiry about their understanding of mindfulness and meditation.
- Patients should be educated about mindfulness as a specific capacity of the mind, with an emphasis on the benefits it offers for managing pain, stress, and various medical conditions; about a favored attitude emphasizing curiosity and nonjudgment; and reassurance it's normal to experience distractions during meditation.
- Instruction should include brief guided practices during the clinical visit and can be followed by recommendations for ongoing practice, handouts, and potential follow-up appointments or referrals to local resources.

Mindfulness-informed Treatment Programs
- Various modalities are discussed including MBSR, MBPM, MBCT, DBT, and ACT; these programs help manage symptoms, reduce stress, improve emotional regulation, and support recovery.
- Each program focuses on different aspects of mindfulness and addresses specific conditions or challenges, targeting stress, chronic pain, depression, emotional regulation, and self-destructive behaviors.

References

1. Priddy SE, Howard MO, Hanley AW, Riquino MR, Friberg-Felsted K, Garland EL. Mindfulness meditation in the treatment of substance use disorders and preventing future relapse: neurocognitive mechanisms and clinical implications. Subst Abuse Rehabil. 2018;9:103–14. https://doi.org/10.2147/SAR.S145201. PMID: 30532612; PMCID: PMC6247953
2. Kabat-Zinn J. Mindfulness-based stress reduction (MBSR). Constructivism in the human sciences. Denton. 2003;8(2):73–83.
3. Pérez-Fernández JI, Salaberria K, Ruiz de Ocenda Á. Mindfulness-based pain management (MBPM) for chronic pain: a randomized clinical trial. Mindfulness. 2022;13:3153–65. https://doi.org/10.1007/s12671-022-02023-1.
4. Sipe WEB, Eisendrath SJ. Mindfulness-based cognitive therapy: theory and practice. Can J Psychiatry. 2012;57(2):63–9. https://doi.org/10.1177/070674371205700202.
5. Linehan MM. Cognitive-behavioral treatment of borderline personality disorder. New York, NY: Guilford Press; 1993.
6. Robins CJ, Chapman AL. Dialectical behavior therapy: current status, recent developments, and future directions. J Personal Disord. 2004;18:73–9.
7. Hayes SC, Luoma JB, Bond FW, Masuda A, Lillis J. Acceptance and commitment therapy: model, processes and outcomes. Psychology Faculty Publications; 2006. p. 101. https://scholarworks.gsu.edu/psych_facpub/101

Chapter 5
Mindfulness in Clinical Care: Settings and Situations

In this overview of the myriad ways that mindfulness training can be a benefit multiplier for effective clinical outcomes, we've covered a basic meditation skill set and some routines and tips on offering that training to our patients. A clinician-friendly summary of "applied" mindfulness programs, media, and other referral resources hopefully raises our collective awareness of these truly useful tools for improving medical care.

As with any modality in medical practice, familiarity with the core content of mindfulness and meditation is best achieved through our own reiteration of mindfulness tactics in clinical situations and settings. The COVID pandemic posed an abrupt challenge for healthcare professionals to immediately and flexibly alter our prior routines around harm reduction through masking, vaccination, and other mitigation tactics. It was a radical example of how quickly we can pivot and incorporate new learning and action into our everyday work.

Fortunately, a "mindful" weaving of mindfulness training into a wide variety of clinical niches and situations need not be driven today by the threat of a world-historical public health emergency. Mindfulness, as we've described, is more a "carrot" than a "stick"—a research-tested capacity that when added and implemented to our current work, improves treatment and wellbeing. We need, and should, not adopt it in response to emergency. Doing so would not be fair to ourselves or toward the practice. To fully harness its potential, healthcare providers need to familiarize themselves with the optimal timing, context, and methods for effectively implementing mindfulness training, which intuitively implies the individual practice of the clinician, as well. To integrate this training into medical care successfully, individual clinicians should possess the basic abilities to teach fundamental mindfulness practices to our patients and to one another (peer-to-peer mentoring being an imperative strategy to foster mindful growth in the clinical workspace). As stated in previous chapters, gaining an understanding of the key similarities, differences, and optimal applications of "applied" mindfulness programs, often available through online or in-person educational courses for individuals and groups, is an important first step in what best fits into one's mindfulness toolbox.

The last chapter took us through a content-based review of the "applied" mindfulness programs. Another approach is to look at some specific clinical settings and situations where mindfulness tactics can make a difference: in preparation for events, in the midst of them, and afterward. Mindfulness practices can be a value-add in these situations and more:

- **Individual clinical consultations and office visits**, particularly as part of an overall physical exam/wellness visit, always keeping the basic tenet in mind that breathing itself is the most basic physiological process and we have an opportunity to instruct patients on it.
- **Medical office and hospital diagnostic and treatment procedures** (phlebotomy, radiologic exams, and pre- and post-surgical situations), where preemptive and acute care training in mindfulness can be used as a stress-adaptive tool, offering a unique capacity for grounding individual or team exercises before, during, and after such situations.
- **Mental healthcare**, weaving mindfulness tactics informally into both the direct interactive counseling work and as a symptoms management and contemplative tool in between visits; including inpatient psychiatric hospital units, intensive/partial hospital/day treatment programs, and residential treatment facilities for psychiatric and substance use disorders; clinical settings that can accommodate group/class teaching for both brief and intermittent/sequenced programs.

Mindfulness practices already have much wider implementation in mental health settings. Our review will focus, then, on primary care and medical specialty visits and procedures.

Addressing the wide variety of particular care settings and situations in which patients and physicians participate could generate a corresponding heap of bespoke mindfulness recipes and tactics. Instead, the intention here is for us to lower the threshold in understanding, effort, and effectiveness. We can foster mindfulness tactics as familiar, even intuitive in stress-inducing healthcare settings, just as most regular meditators find themselves doing in the course of other challenging moments in our daily lives—traffic jams, meeting presentations, project deadlines, up at night with a crying infant or waiting on a late-arriving teen. Regardless of the type of stress, health-related or not, we can guide our patients toward a few clear, straightforward, and effective practices that can be easily adapted to many settings and circumstances—rather than a dense "rulebook" of self-awareness recipes. We can focus on understanding and teaching these four accessible practices, each with a slight variation in intention and benefit, yet beneficial in application to that variety of settings and events.

Mindful Tools for Clinical Situations: Four Core Tactics

Mindfulness practices, to reiterate, do not eliminate our inborn threat response (nor should they). However some brief, easily applicable tactics in mindful self-calming and stress management can ease that initial burst of tension and allow for better preparation for an effective visit and/or interaction. Here are four broad categories of tactics to consider teaching patients in preparation for their office visits:

1. **Mindful Breathing:** The core technique of mindful breathing—observing the sensation of breathing to build facility in observation while limiting additional judgment or added thought, especially in the inevitable losing and regaining of that action—is the first and arguably the most important among the four care tactics.
   - Focusing on the breath with the mind's eye is an ideal method for learning to meditate, such as a setting (focused attention with the mind) and anchor or target (the breath) being **always present**—"school's always open."
   - It is a simple, yet foundational example of the **inevitability of change in our human experience**; no in-and-out breath sequence is the same, and no observing of that sequence ever stays the same, and anxiety and judgment will arise even toward these minor unfamiliar circumstances. That reality makes it an **ideal practice ground for losing and regaining attention in the background of a novel human experience.**
   - Furthermore, breath observation routinely **self-generates calming** and thus reinforces **a sense of agency** over one's momentary physical state, however, fraught.
   - As has been shown, training in this basic focusing of attention on the breath and observing its natural rhythm is **not complicated**.
   - Finally, its utility and benefits are truly **portable**.

   These attributes as both an entry path to mindfulness more broadly and as a routinely therapeutic response in terms of adoption to acute, momentary stress make training in basic breath meditation an essential tactic, one that other momentary mindful practices can be built upon.
2. **Scanning:** This is a tactic that builds on the basic targeting of the particular sensation and location in breath meditation to involve shifting our observation sequentially from one target of personal experience to another. In general, mindfulness training via meditation, as well as in mindful movement practices, a key step in training, after gaining facility with the breath as a target, is building familiarity with flexibly directing our awareness. Mindful awareness, whether in meditation or in daily life, is a capacity of mind that can be operated like a camera, focusing and directing attention on individual phenomena of our current experience, like the breath, heartbeat, or back pain, and out to the "landscape" of the physical, emotional, and thought phenomena of the moment, in part or whole. That capacity can be directed outward to the perception of the local space around the individual, and even out beyond.

Applying this aspect of flexibility and direction of awareness to the clinical setting is sensible and valuable. This technique involves directing awareness to the body and systematically scanning it for any sensations or areas of tension or discomfort. Patients are taught to proceed through the sequence with curiosity rather than critique and judgment and to inevitably notice what areas generate excess judgment anyway. This practice can help individuals become more attuned to and adaptive to normal bodily sensations, as well as any heightened anxiety-related sensations. With practice, one can better understand and regulate their physical responses, reducing unnecessary worry or anxious thoughts. Noticing areas of tension or discomfort often spontaneously leads to some release through deep breathing and relaxation techniques, further promoting a sense of calm and well-being. Some variations here include:

- **Body scan meditation** simply involves moving the target of one's mindful awareness, up or down the physical self from the experience of one's breath to, say, feet, then legs, then waist and upward, or scalp and downward, covering the full body of somatic experience.
- For many, **a "combined" tactic** is helpful—of attending to the breath on inhalation, and then directing attention on each exhalation to the sequential bodily targets. A kind of "**gathering**" then "**directing**" awareness in imagination parallels the calming of sequential breaths.
- A slightly broader variation on the body scan, which could be called a "**self**" scan (or "**me**" scan), involves sequential targets of awareness beyond physical phenomena to a full attending to body, emotions, thoughts, and then a full opening to self-in-the-moment. Using the "gathering and directing" tactic, noted above, the sequence involves a breath or more (inhaling to noting the breath, then exhaling to these targets) on bodily sensations; then moving to emotional tone (often located in the chest or heart area); then to observing prominent thoughts in the moment; then a final breath or more pulling attention out to the self in whole—body, heart, and head—in this moment. This broader, systematic practice of attending sequentially through not just somatic experience, but the associated emotional, thought/ruminative, and then a "full self" experiential view is especially effective as a rescue tactic for those in acute emotional distress, such as panic events, intense anger/dysphoria, craving, and urges toward craving self-harm or suicidal ideation.

Whether of the physical realm only, or of a fuller survey of all inner experience, this scanning practice is valuable in addressing acute suffering and in grounding individuals in better momentary self-awareness and self-control. It has wide applicability in a variety of medical settings and situations.

3. **Visualization:** This is an imaginal tactic, which can also be paired with mindful breathing. It is used regularly in working with phobias; for example, using imagination to mentally rehearse and gradually desensitize to the feared situation such as driving over a bridge, prior to and preparing for subsequent, direct exposure to the event. Visualization techniques can include creating a detailed mental picture of an anticipated event, incorporating remembered or anticipated sights,

sounds, and physical sensations, and proceeding through the event in imagination. "Imaginal Rehearsal Therapy" (IRT) is another term of art for this practice, which has also shown benefit in veterans populations to address flashbacks and night terrors associated with PTSD.

It can operate beneficially as a basic "run through" of an event. In addition, the visualization/imaginal "script" can also include creating and mentally rehearsing successful or preferred outcomes. This can be a simple, brief "snapshot" of oneself as calm and effective in the waiting and consulting room or of the feeling after a positive meeting with a clinician. For others, a visualized, more granular "walk-through" rehearsal of the event can be done, from travel to the waiting room to a beneficial interaction and satisfied completion. Through visualization, patients picture themselves interacting smoothly with healthcare providers and receiving clear and helpful information.

4. **Gratitude/Compassion Meditation:** The inclusion of brief meditations on opening to the aspirational states of **gratitude and compassion** can also be valuable in medical settings. These practices focus less on a momentary awareness of one's state and instead work to generate and/or access one's positive, aspirational feelings, to the extent they can be accessed in the midst of discomfort. Gratitude meditation involves **focusing on feelings of appreciation and acknowledging the positive aspects of one's healthcare experience**, including the opportunity to receive medical care, the knowledge and expertise of healthcare professionals, and the support of loved ones, shifting the mindset from anxiety and worry to a more positive outlook. Compassion meditation, on the other hand, is **cultivating empathy toward oneself, fellow patients, healthcare providers, and staff**, while acknowledging one's own fears and anxieties.

Cultivating gratitude fosters a positive and supportive atmosphere for the patient/clinician relationship. Patients who express gratitude tend to feel more satisfied with their healthcare experience. Gratitude acknowledges the efforts and expertise of the healthcare team. It can promote a sense of mutual respect and understanding, leading to better communication and collaboration between patients and caregivers.

Cultivating compassion can help patients develop a kind and understanding attitude toward themselves, particularly during times of illness, pain, or vulnerability. Self-compassion allows patients to be gentle and patient with themselves, acknowledging their own suffering without judgment or self-criticism.

These practices can help shift the predominant mindset from anxiety and worry to a more positive outlook. The opening to these positive states of mind is meant to occur in parallel, in the same "field" of mind, rather than as a superficially concocted state to replace, suppress, or "bypass" other, perhaps uncomfortable emotional states that may also be present. As such, there are some potential risks associated with trying to generate gratitude and compassion when it is not genuinely present or accessible within oneself. There is a risk of feeling the aspirational state is inauthentic, insincere; or that underlying suffering is to be ignored or judged as unacceptable.

The favored direction is to "open to" images or feelings of compassion and gratitude, and then observe the effect in heart and mind—rather than a forced sense of "play-acting" at a state of mind. When accessible, these meditations can foster a sense of resilience, optimism, and collaborative trust in the healthcare process.

As noted, there are many variations on these and associated mindful practices that can be helpful for patients across medical settings and situations. The four foundational examples covered—breath meditation, scanning practice, visualization, and gratitude/compassion meditation—represent a useful, easily conveyed set of mindful tools for physicians to educate our patients about. There is shared benefit in the clinical relationship, and in some particular medical settings and situations.

The Office Visit

Clinical consultations in the office setting are an essential, critical aspect of healthcare delivery, providing an opportunity for physicians to connect with our patients and provide individualized care. Yet this basic "unit" of care also represents an uncertain and anxiety-provoking event for many individuals. Patients may react to a sense of minimal control, and feel vulnerable and at the mercy of healthcare professionals. The uncertainty surrounding the purpose and progress of the visit, the potential outcomes, and procedures or treatments that may result or occur can contribute to our patients' potential sense of unease. Valid concerns about wait times, compressed face-to-face visit times, and financial implications can further color the overall experience.

Some of these stresses of office-based care are inevitable aspects of the human condition and the threat and reality of medical illness. Unfortunately, other stressful aspects are endemic to contemporary healthcare. In all, we ask a lot of our patients in tolerating and adapting to the unique circumstances of the clinical situation. Incorporating mindfulness techniques into clinical consultations can be incredibly beneficial for both physicians and patients alike, specifically in that task of tolerance and adaptation—of holding the stress, and being more present and aware as an effective participant in the doctor/patient dyad.

A useful way to walk through the opportunities for mindfulness utilization in this setting is to "slow down the video"—looking at the components of the event in a granular way as a set of sequences our patients pass through in any office visit.

Pre-Visit: As any (or all) of us who have been on the other end of the stethoscope can understand, the initial flow of experience associated with the office visit is its anticipation. The mere trigger of a note on the calendar, or more likely currently, a text or email reminder from a healthcare provider of an upcoming scheduled visit, can set off interior alarms. Besides the suffering of that tension, "downfield" problems can result from the stress, including distraction from remembering or documenting essential data for the visit to being late for or even missing the visit. Negative impacts on the quality of our care become more likely.

Incorporating any or all of the four core practices into clinical consultations can benefit patients prior to the office visit.

- By practicing techniques such as **focused breathing and body scan meditation,** patients can feel more relaxed and at ease heading into the office and then the consulting room.
- Encouraging patients to use **visualization tactics** can be part of a visit prep information package. Each visualization segment need not be elaborate; patients can be directed to some initial relaxation breathing, then a rehearsal in mind for fruitful clinical interaction, as noted above. Such brief visualizations can proceed through:
    - **Home preparation** (adequate time for travel, a few major questions/concerns considered and documented, etc.).
    - Initial **waiting room** interactions, including mindful tactics in management of anxiety re: waiting, uncertainty.
    - The **office visit** itself includes interactions with physician, NP/PA, RN, and other staff).
    - **Resolution**/regrouping/travel home—including post-visit documentation of treatment recommendations/changes and reflection on the event.
- **Gratitude/Compassion meditation** is, as has been noted, a potentially helpful frame-of-mind modification exercise, especially as it may bring to awareness conditioned tensions around negativity, pessimism, and even catastrophic, worst-case-scenario ruminations based in past health crises or traumatic past interactions with healthcare professionals. Again, this exercise is not meant to encroach on or replace individual spiritual beliefs or practices. Nevertheless, "sitting with" the felt state of feeling grateful for an expectation of aid, and of empathy for one's own state of suffering can counter preset, reflexive conditioning about "things going wrong."

As the core tactics are meant to reduce tension prior to clinical interaction, some teaching or resource access would be helpful at the outset. This can be done via offering media links to these practices along with text/email reminders of the upcoming visit. A handout given with the usual administrative paperwork that provides a "walk through" of brief breath and/or scanning practice can be effective. Some office settings may have the space to create a quiet corner or room for brief pre-visit practice or reflection.

A fruitful potential use of smartphone technology is to incorporate guided versions of these core practices into applications, including the patient-centered apps now widely utilized by medical groups for visit scheduling, lab result reporting, and communication with the office and clinicians. Finally, as will be covered in more detail later, a medical staff that models calm self-awareness through their own familiarity with mindfulness reinforces the opportunity offered for individuals (Table 5.1).

Table 5.1 Pre-visit mindfulness techniques

- Focused breathing: Reducing pre-visit anxiety and improving relaxation
- Body/ "self" scan: Sequential grounding in current somatic, emotional and thought state of the moment
- Visualization: Mentally rehearsing the visit for reduced stress and better preparedness
- Gratitude/compassion meditation: Cultivating positive states to counteract negativity and pessimism

Into the visit: Anxiety for most patients amplifies with entry into the office waiting area, checking in with office staff, and completing forms about payment and symptom checklists. The uncertainty of the waiting follows. The visualization rehearsal work done prior hopefully softens the anxiety and frustration that can be generated; breath training and scan exercises are most helpful in addressing momentary uncertainty and anxiety.

It peaks with the office staff invitation into the clinical suite. Physicians and patients alike know the "gauntlet": the "rooming," taking of vital signs and other information, then commonly a solitary wait in a sanitized but somewhat sterile, often less-than-welcome environment. The breath training and scan exercises can help here, which could prompt to patients who have been already instructed on their use. Otherwise, time allowing, it can be an opportune moment to briefly introduce basic breath practice, which also helps familiarize patients to staff and the clinic environment. For many clinicians, especially in psychiatry and psychotherapy work, an initial moment of shared "tuning in" via simultaneous, brief, meditation sets a tone not only of mutual intention to be "peak-present" for the work but a therapeutic collaboration, as well.

For other patients, a couple of breaths with self-compassion in mind for this unusual moment in the patient's day can lower the tension level. A few more with gratitude as the imagined state can pivot experience from threat to anticipation of that collaboration, and of being attended to with competence and care.

For patients who have experienced physical, emotional, and/or sexual trauma and suffer from PTSD, the confined spaces of a waiting room and especially an exam room can feel intensely threatening and trigger overwhelming responses such as panic attacks and flashbacks. While it is a routine aspect of PTSD treatment to help patients entrain self-calming tactics, including breath meditation and scanning, some individuals may nevertheless not have those skills yet or are overwhelmed enough to be distracted from using those tools. Physicians, staff, and chaperones can be sensitive to these emergent moments and be able to offer brief, shared, guided breath tactics and scanning. Facilities with these allow for a truly therapeutic intervention at the moment, as well as help create an environment of safety and support for the clinical interview.

The physical examination is perhaps the apex of the clinical interaction in terms of an optimum placed on calm awareness for both patient and clinician. Even informal modeling of slow, steady breathing on the part of us clinicians as we run the familiar sequence of examination tactics. Patients familiar with mindful tactics may operate intuitively in the same way, modeling calm for a harried, distracted physician rushing through visit.

The sequence of the standard physical exam is so very familiar to physicians that we may not realize it is not necessarily so for our patients. Maintaining a calm dialogue to signal intentions before each tactile event in the examination may seem self-explanatory. Yet, a brief "rehearsal"/ modeled visualization of the sequence of assessments can be helpful to patients, especially those who express worry or appear tense. We show care and respect in a brief "here's what I plan to examine next" contracting, particularly when involving instrumentation (otoscopes, tongue depressors, and reflex hammers) or in approaching areas reported as tender or of concern. Eye contact and a slow breath in preparation is a mundane but fruitful example of inviting—and employing—mindfulness in vulnerable moments for our patients.

Vulnerable moments: Encouraging and modeling mindfulness can be particularly useful during the most vulnerable aspects of the physical exam, as they are consented to. These moments obviously include examination of genital areas, breast, pelvic, and prostate exams. Reinforcing breath and body scan tactics can help our patients manage the discomfort, anxiety, or vulnerability they may experience. A brief visualized "walk-through" of the exam components with descriptions of tactile cues (then reiterating each during the exam—"this is when you'll feel a little bit of a cold sensation," for example) is, again, mostly a second-nature action for experienced clinicians. Yet it is a simple, powerful way to impart a sense of awareness of the interactive moment while gathering data. It can also, unfortunately, drop away in this era of compressed time and expectations.

Of course, just like the examination itself, offering patients help with mindfulness tactics should be contracted for rather than imposed. One notable alternative to practices that encourage sharpened but calm attention to the moment is when a patient expresses direct concern that "tuning-in" actually amplifies anxiety. In such cases, suggesting an alternative visualization—visualizing a peaceful place or calming image, for instance—can be more comforting (Table 5.2).

Post-visit: The preparatory mindful exercise in imaginal "rehearsal" can positively impact this phase of the entire office visit experience. Especially in the situation of new and difficult information conveyed in the office visit, patients can nevertheless exit the office feeling flooded in thoughts and emotions. It's natural for many individuals to make that exit briskly and mindlessly; yet encouraging patients to take a few moments to sit quietly afterward, whether back in the waiting room, or prior to travel back home, is medical practice at its mindful best.

Patients can sit briefly in observation of experience just completed, which can run the gamut from relief to uncertainty to fear, sadness, and grievance. The fuller "self" scan can be a framework to observe any thoughts, emotions, or physical sensations that arise. **It can be helpful for patients to briefly document the state and**

Table 5.2 Mindfulness during the visit

- Anxiety amplification: Addressing heightened tension from waiting room to examination
- Mindful breathing/scanning: Techniques to manage discomfort and vulnerability during examination
- Visualization for vulnerable moments: Mentally preparing for sensitive exam aspects
- Alternative visualization: For patients where focused attention increases anxiety

any instructions, while the memory of the office visit is fresh in mind. Pithy note-taking works, as does encouraging those with a smartphone to leave themselves a quick voice-to-text of the visit.

The emotional impact of a medical visit, particularly if it involves receiving distressing news or undergoing a stressful procedure, may contribute to distraction or reduced attention. Recommending a few moments of mindful breath observation to moderate an intense state is sensible prior to, say, driving home.

Patients often benefit from having a family member or friend accompany them for medical office visits. The emotional support is obvious, and the "second set of ears" can help validate and reality-test information conveyed. This is also an opportunity for a shared mindful practice experience, if the companion is willing to participate. By engaging in mindfulness practices together, such as breathing exercises or body scans, patients and their companions can create a shared sense of calm and presence. While meditation is an interior experience in practice, practicing with others is uniquely helpful, as many meditators who gather to practice on retreats and in scheduled group settings can attest. The shared sense of support and mutual intention found in those experiences is also potent when used in this circumstance.

In sum, the "routine" office visit, when unpacked into its component moments, reveals a series of events that can benefit from mindful tactics. Improved self-regulation of anxiety and uncertainty generates less suffering for our patients, and a greater likelihood of accurate assessment and clear communication. The "core four" tactics reviewed—breath meditation, scanning (body, self), visualization, and gratitude/compassion meditation—are straightforward to teach, making them ideal to fold into our patients' "tool kit" of self-help capacities (Table 5.3).

We can and should employ them—routinely—to optimize our office visits.

Clinical Procedures

While the sequence of events that make up a patient's experience of a routine office visit has its predictable nodal points of potential tension, modern healthcare has less routine and yet more potentially intense events for us and our patients to navigate: clinical procedures. These include diagnostic procedures, such as phlebotomy, imaging (radiography, ultrasound, mammogram CT, MRI), and the varieties of endoscopic procedures. As medical technology has developed, many intensive, at times invasive therapeutic procedures have migrated to same-day events and settings; these include outpatient surgeries, hemodialysis, radiotherapies, and chemotherapies. That migration can lead us to underestimate the sense of risk and threat

Table 5.3 Post-visit mindfulness

- Reflecting on the visit: Using mindfulness to process and document the experience
- Ensuring safety: Mindful breathing before driving or other tasks post-visit
- Shared mindfulness practices: Engaging companions in mindfulness for mutual support

Clinical Procedures

that patients can experience through the pre-, peri-, and post-procedure components. While most younger adult patients accept outpatient procedures as standard and common, older adults can ironically perceive more risk rather than less, with a latent sense that such events should require the relatively increased safety of a hospital environment.

The same "core four" mindfulness tactics may be fruitfully used by patients (and taught by clinicians) in the variety of procedures noted. Here are some selected examples of applications.

Phlebotomy: The blood draw is one of the most common procedures in medicine. While mundane for many, it also can draw the most intense phobic reactions in some patients, at times driven by early conditioning of and association to childhood illness and/or painful/traumatic "sticks." The uniqueness of seeing one's own blood can also play a role in phobic reactions during blood draws. Blood is an integral part of our body, and witnessing it outside of its usual context can be unsettling for some individuals. The sight of blood can evoke feelings of vulnerability or disgust, and this visceral reaction can intensify anxiety during the procedure. The fear of needles (trypanophobia) is a common phobia that can be triggered by the sight, thought, or anticipation of a needle puncturing the skin. The perception of pain associated with needle insertion can further amplify this fear response. Individuals may also have a fear of fainting, often associated with the sight of blood or the act of having blood drawn, which adds another layer of anxiety to the experience, as the anxiety includes a fear of public loss of bodily control and secondary shame over the event.

Mindfulness techniques can be incredibly beneficial in managing phlebotomy. Breathing exercises (first, directed relaxation/belly breathing, then mindful observation of the breath) can be employed to help patients relax and reduce feelings of apprehension. By taking slow, deliberate breaths, individuals activate their body's natural relaxation response, lowering heart rate and blood pressure. Scanning pre-, peri-, and post-"stick" allows for framing the event in an "observation" mode, parallel to (modifying but not replacing) the "immersion" mode that the anxious moment drives. This is also a good way to work with patients with known difficulties with phlebotomy to prepare via visualization practice (best before arrival at the laboratory center)—walking through the sequence of events and feelings, attending in imagination to the reactions that can occur and even rehearsing alternative, successful scenarios. For some with truly intense phobic reactions, the recommendation for visualizing an alternative, calming image is appropriate. Finally, many patients with even minor tension around this procedure have their own "horror stories" about a particularly difficult "stick," the phlebotomist missing multiple times and generating pain. (Physicians have our own reciprocal tales about "impossible" blood draw attempts on patients from our training years, and the helplessness that can ensue!) Gratitude/compassion meditation, while sounding ironic, can nevertheless counter the prevailing anticipatory negativity with an aspiration for the phlebotomist's skillful work.

Imaging: Some tension over imaging procedures dates back to the first radiographs, despite their ubiquity in modern medical care. Beyond the concerns about short and long-term risks of ionizing radiation, the procedure generates some of the familiar sensory triggers and aspects we note above. Radiology suites are a relatively impersonal, sterile setting, with intimidating equipment and unusual, unfamiliar sounds. There is the prospect of requests to hold physical positions that are unusual and sometimes painful. The expectation of personal exposure and lack of privacy can heighten vulnerability over body image.

All four of the core "acute use" tactics are helpful here, in ways similar to procedures described above. Breath and scanning tactics are effective in the midst of any imaging procedure. Especially with imaging that involves longer time periods, such as MRI, encouraging pre-event visualization of the sequence—gowning, positioning on the table (back support, application of protective ear plugs, etc.), then the scanning sequence—can reduce the anxiety involved and arguably lead to less complications and better imaging outcomes. The rehearsal can be done via a recollection of a prior MRI by the patient, or if a first time in the device, by the ordering physician in preparation, via media, or informally by friends and family with experience. In the case of CT with contrast, rehearsal can include awareness of and anticipation for unusual sensory experiences, including quick spreading, then resolution of perceived warmth or cooling; a temporary metallic taste; and the possibility of nausea or infiltration of the contrast into the subcutaneous soft tissues. Any of these unusual experiences can be amplified by surprise and secondary fear; and they can be moderated with some careful pre-event informing and brief rehearsal, as well as reminder to use breath tactics throughout the procedure.

MRI also merits special mention for its other anxiety-provoking features to prepare for. The tight space is an obvious claustrophobia trigger for some. The unusual abrupt changes in sound can be difficult to tolerate, especially for those not prepared to face them. Finally, the expectation of holding still through all of that lest the result be fouled up by inadvertent motion or other artifact looms over the whole affair. Besides a patient's own mindful adaptation, with basic breath meditation in the midst of the scanning being the most important tool, having imaging technicians familiar with these tactics can be a true value-add in radiology departments, offering some brief breath practice at the outset of scanning, and regular audio contact with the patient throughout the procedure.

Endoscopy: The remarkable utility of endoscopy/arthroscopy in all its forms has truly revolutionized care in a host of specialties, including GI, OB/GYN ENT, urology, neurology, orthopedics, and other surgical subspecialties. Yet we cannot underplay the stress of such procedures, involving anxiety over discomfort, loss of control, and vulnerability. That a subset of these procedures access areas of the body deemed private and even may have associations with trauma should amplify our awareness of and caution about the procedures' psychological impacts; however, important the clinical knowledge gained. Those "process" stressors occur in the setting of underlying worry about results and the prospect of distressing diagnostic findings.

The "four core" tactics do not need further extensive reiteration here. For clinicians, identifying ideal ways to include teaching and training is key. That can include in-office discussion, a separate video or telehealth contact, or directing to media sources that both describe the sequences in the procedure and also specific information on using mindful tactics to prepare for (using visualization/rehearsal) and tolerate (using breath and scanning) the procedure.

One unique concern that is important to prepare for is the generally beneficial use of a mix of sedative medications for the procedure. As this represents a rather abrupt shift in consciousness, for some individuals anxious reactions that loss of control may override the calming benefits. Furthermore, the amnestic effects associated with midazolam (an ultra-short-acting benzodiazepine in routine use for such procedures) can cause a loss of memory for not just the procedure (anterograde amnesia) but occasionally also retrograde amnesia—a loss of memory of events occurring for some minutes prior to the dose being administered intravenously. The mechanism is poorly understood, with the possibility of an impact on initial memory storage. In any event, both of these effects can result in patients waking up into confusion and agitation about their location, that the procedure has been completed and even the circumstances of minutes prior to sedation. This moment can be anticipated and managed by pre-procedure education and preparation on the part of staff, adding this possible outcome to the visualization rehearsal, and a support person at bedside for reassurance and a prompt for mindful breathing tactics.

Ongoing/Sequenced Treatments (hemodialysis, chemotherapy, radiotherapy): The core mindful tactics reviewed above are also well-suited for these repetitive, challenging treatments. All involve managing and tolerating the waxing and waning physical aspects of these medical procedures, and the emotional variability that comes with uncertainty over treatment effect. Mindfulness allows individuals to cultivate a nonreactive and accepting attitude toward their experiences, helping them navigate the challenges more effectively and find moments of calm and peace amidst the treatment process.

The Mindful Medical Office: Implementation and Monitoring

Incorporating a suite of mindfulness practices and tactics into all clinical routines in patient visits and procedures could include some initial education of new patients into the clinic or practice about the basics covered above, benefits, and opportunities for further learning. This can be done by clinical staff with training, a designated staff specialist in teaching mindfulness, or via social media (practice website video/audio clips). Besides the usual signage that covers privacy notices, patients' rights, and hygiene policies, educational posters on exercise and nutrition may be augmented by brief breath meditation training information—helpful training in that setting and moment.

Monitoring the effectiveness of a mindfulness program for patient care helps ensure that the program is meeting its intended goals and improving patient outcomes. Clear and measurable goals for the program should be set at the outset. One way to monitor the effectiveness of a mindfulness program is to use pre- and post-program assessments to track changes in patient outcomes over time. This might include measures of mental health symptoms, quality of life, and mindfulness-related constructs such as awareness and nonjudgment.

In addition, it may be useful to track changes in healthcare utilization, such as the frequency of hospitalizations or emergency department visits, to assess the program's impact on healthcare costs. It may be useful to compare changes in patient outcomes to a control group or to normative data to assess the program's impact relative to what might be expected in the absence of the program.

Another important aspect of monitoring and evaluating the effectiveness of a mindfulness program is to gather feedback from patients and healthcare providers to provide valuable information about the program's strengths and weaknesses, as well as areas for improvement. This can be done through surveys or focus groups. In addition, monitoring patient engagement with structured programs (e.g., attendance at sessions and completion of homework assignments) can help identify barriers to participation and inform program modifications to improve patient engagement and adherence (Tables 5.4 and 5.5).

Please see the appendix of this book for a multitude of measures that can be employed in the clinical setting.

Implementing and Monitoring a Mindful Medical Office

In Summary: Applying Mindfulness at the Bedside

This chapter is meant to illuminate the ways mindful awareness can be applied across the spectrum of direct clinical interactions. We started with clarifying the range of tactics, reinforcing the "core four tactics for us to become familiar with and facile in educating our patients about. The four—mindful breathing, scanning practice (body scan, body/emotions/thought "self" scan), visualization/rehearsal, and aspirational (gratitude/compassion) practice—have distinct circumstances and benefits that will become more familiar and intuitive to us as clinicians, but only with our own intentional practice in implementing them.

That developing knowledge of the positive impact of mindfulness practices, and the resulting tendency toward weaving them into our everyday clinical work, certainly is more likely with some reminders to include them in the workplace. They

Table 5.4 Integrating mindfulness into the image of the clinic

- Initial patient education: Introduce mindfulness basics, benefits, and further learning opportunities
- Staff training and resources: Train clinical staff or designate a mindfulness specialist
- Use of social media and signage: Leverage practice websites, videos, audio clips, and educational posters

In Summary: Applying Mindfulness at the Bedside

Table 5.5 Setting clear goals for mindfulness programs

• Measurable objectives: Establish specific, measurable outcomes for the mindfulness program • Patient outcome tracking: Use pre- and post-assessments to monitor mental health, quality of life, and mindfulness skills • Healthcare utilization metrics: Track changes in hospitalizations or emergency visits to assess cost impact	

Feedback collection and analysis	Program evaluation and improvement
• **Patient and provider feedback:** Gather insights through surveys or focus groups to evaluate program strengths and weaknesses • **Monitoring patient engagement:** Track attendance, homework completion, and participation in mindfulness sessions • **Identifying barriers:** Use engagement data to identify and address barriers to program adherence	• **Comparative analysis:** Compare patient outcomes with control groups or normative data for relative impact assessment • **Continuous improvement:** Use feedback and engagement data to refine and enhance the mindfulness program • **Tailoring approaches:** Adjust program elements based on specific patient needs and clinic capabilities

are much more likely, however, to take hold if we personally engage in them ourselves and with our healthcare peers and partners. The next chapter will explore that corner of mindfulness in medicine: leveraging and implementing our own mindfulness practices as a professional and personal benefit.

Key Points

Mindfulness Training for Clinical Outcomes Enhancement
- Mindfulness training can significantly improve clinical outcomes by offering a basic meditation skill set and providing strategies for implementing this training with patients—promoting improved treatment and well-being.
- It is important for healthcare professionals to become familiar with core mindfulness and meditation concepts and be equipped to teach fundamental mindfulness practices to patients and colleagues, integrating mindfulness into various clinical settings, in both routine and acute/emergent situations.
- "Applied" mindfulness programs, available through various educational courses for individuals and groups, should be explored and understood to optimize their applications in healthcare settings.

Mindful Tools for Clinical Situations: Four Core Tactics
- Mindfulness practices—mindful breathing, scanning, visualization, and gratitude/compassion meditation—are accessible and adaptable to various medical settings and situations and can be valuable tools in various clinical situations.
- Mindful breathing involves observing the sensation of breathing to improve focus and relaxation. It is a foundational practice that can be easily integrated into daily life.
- Scanning is a technique that helps individuals systematically shift their awareness from one target of experience to another, enhancing self-awareness and adaptability.

- Visualization, used to mentally rehearse events or create positive outcomes, can alleviate anxiety and improve patients' mental readiness for medical procedures.
- Gratitude and compassion meditation can foster positive mindsets and enhance the patient–provider relationship. They promote empathy, self-compassion, and resilience.

The Office Visit: Enhancing Patient Experience through Mindfulness
- Clinical consultations in the office setting can be anxiety-inducing for patients, and mindfulness techniques can be employed to improve their experience. Mindfulness training can optimize routine office visits by improving patient self-regulation, reducing suffering, and enhancing communication between patients and clinicians.
- Patients can benefit from practicing mindfulness before, during, and after office visits to reduce stress and enhance their capacity to cope with medical procedures and uncertainty.
- Companions accompanying patients can also participate in mindfulness practices, creating a shared sense of calm and support.

Clinical Procedures
- Clinical procedures in modern healthcare encompass various diagnostic and therapeutic techniques, including phlebotomy, imaging (radiography, ultrasound, mammogram CT, MRI), and endoscopic procedures—events that can generate anxiety and stress for patients.
- Mindfulness techniques, including breathing exercises, visualization, and gratitude/compassion meditation, can help patients manage anxiety and discomfort during procedures like phlebotomy.
- Ongoing treatments like hemodialysis, chemotherapy, and radiotherapy can benefit from mindfulness practices in managing physical and emotional challenges.

The Mindful Medical Office: Implementation and Monitoring
- Integrating mindfulness practices into clinical routines involves educating patients about the benefits and opportunities for mindfulness learning, either by clinical staff, specialists, or through social media.
- Monitoring the effectiveness of a mindfulness program includes setting clear goals, conducting pre- and post-program assessments, tracking changes in patient outcomes, assessing the impact on healthcare utilization and costs, and identifying barriers to participation to improve patient engagement and adherence.

Chapter 6
The Mindful Healthcare Professional

In this overview of mindfulness and its application across the spectrum of healthcare, we began by broadly defining the capacity of mindfulness and its training in meditative practices. We focused on the neuropsychological "backstory" and summarized the evidence for its profound benefits. The last two chapters have framed out varieties of mindful tactics, exercises, and programming that currently exist to benefit our patients. We then moved to a review of the particular medical settings and situations in which these tactics can play a beneficial role for those patients.

The spotlight thus far has emphasized mindfulness as a patient-centered value and identified the range of meditative practices that can cultivate that valuable capacity. We've also touched on how individual practice can improve the doctor–patient relationship, as well as clinical performance, be it one-on-one in the clinic or as a team in the trauma bay. The added value for individuals in our care includes their reduction in overt suffering, adaptation to our diagnostic and treatment routines, and collaboration with us in providing effective healthcare.

Yet patient care is at its core a dyad—a relationship. The outcome of our work benefits from, if not depends upon, the mutual trust, shared values, and partnership in that dyad. Our participation in alliance-building is an aspiration introduced to us from the outset of all forms and settings of healthcare training. It is reinforced throughout our training pathways and then inevitably cultivated through experience in our ongoing, subsequent work. However competent we caregivers are in our role, we are individuals participating with others in a shared goal. Mindfulness, as has been reiterated, can help our patients participate optimally in that relationship.

But what about the other participant(s) in that dyad? What might mindfulness do for us as healthcare professionals? The next chapters will provide an overview of the types, benefits, and implementation of mindfulness practices for individual physicians, nurses, and allied healthcare providers. We will examine how mindfulness can benefit larger sets: medical teams, hospitals, and hospital systems. We will also look at the prospects for integrating mindfulness training as a core feature of medical and other healthcare training programs. As a practical, trainable capacity with direct benefits for our well-being, as well as in improving our performance, mindfulness arguably deserves a foundational place in all healthcare training curricula.

To gather an appreciation for mindfulness in medicine, it makes sense to first do some looking around, both outward and inward. Surveying the landscape, the acceleration of change in how healthcare is provided is dizzying in pace, content, and expectations. Adaptation to this surge is a challenge that mindfulness practices can help all of us with. It's also worthwhile, if possibly uncomfortable, to briefly take a look in the mirror. Individuals who choose healthcare as a career in general identify with qualities and aspirations that are ideally beneficial to society, as well as ourselves as individuals. Yet these same temperamental qualities can generate blind spots in our work, both in quality and our fulfillment, that mindfulness practices can help us minimize and adapt to. We'll explore those "interior" dynamics as well. Before we summarize some basic recommendations and suggestions, we'll stare down the healthcare professional's biggest risk: "burnout." First, we look outward.

The Current State of Healthcare

Medicine is a challenging, fulfilling profession. It provides a professional/career "ecosystem" like no other in contemporary society. It is and has ever been an exciting but demanding one.

As caregivers, we've always faced numerous challenges on a daily basis. They range from the demanding workload and ongoing learning curve in maintaining clinical excellence, to our individual challenges in sustaining our own physical and emotional wellbeing in the midst of working with the suffering of others. It's the job, regardless of our age or circumstances.

Yet even before the world-historical pandemic, but especially since, the medical profession has experienced a remarkable surge in stressors [1], with mounting workloads, technological complexities, administrative burdens, and emotional pressures. The COVID-19 pandemic undoubtedly served as a prime catalyst in pushing the boundaries and expectations of our endurance and adaptation to unprecedented levels. It highlights the urgent need for support, resilience, and systemic changes within our industry.

- The ever-increasing **workload** [2] poses a tremendous challenge. The rising demand for healthcare services, coupled with a shortage of medical professionals, has resulted in heavy patient caseloads and longer working hours. Physicians often find ourselves stretched thin, trying to provide quality care while managing numerous cases simultaneously. The sheer volume of patients to be seen, coupled with the complexity of cases, leaves little room for downtime or breaks. We often face the dilemma of balancing a need for thorough, quality care with pressures to meet productivity targets. This workload pressure compromises patient care as fatigue and burnout can generate struggles in empathy and errors in diagnosis and treatment [3].

- **Bureaucratic burdens** [4] have become another source of mounting stress. "Big data" via electronic health records (EHRs) promised to improve coordination of care, enhance clinical decision making and thus healthcare outcomes and research. But the reality for many of us is information overload. Extra effort is needed to sift through irrelevant or redundant data, making it difficult to extract meaningful insights and identify critical information in a timely manner. Poorly designed interfaces, complex workflows, and interoperability challenges across different healthcare systems necessitate extra time in gaining facility with new or legacy data systems. Clinicians spend excessive time navigating the EHR interface instead of engaging directly with our patients. Frustration, reduced efficiency, and potential errors become inevitable. The necessary but encroaching privacy/HIPAA concerns around sensitive patient information—that data are a prime target for unauthorized access, data breaches, and potential misuse—only add more bureaucratic tension in maintaining patient trust while complying with legal and regulatory requirements. Physicians are also increasingly burdened with navigating complex insurance systems, completing documentation, and managing billing and coding requirements. This burden has grown exponentially, diverting precious time and energy away from patient care. These bureaucratic demands generate disconnection from our core mission of providing quality care.
- The increasing **amount and complexity of medical knowledge** [5] is an underappreciated source of stress for healthcare professionals. As we pride ourselves on our intellectual capacities (more on that below), healthcare professionals may underplay the challenge of keeping up with the rapidly expanding breadth of research, technologies, and treatment options constantly emerging. That explosive pace—a recently reported data point is that the sheer amount of medical knowledge "doubles in less than three months"—makes the task of staying current with these advancements improbable and overwhelming for physicians already managing demanding workloads. The complexity of diagnosing and treating patients has also intensified, with cases often presenting with multiple comorbidities, intricate medical histories, and problematic socioeconomic circumstances impacting care options. Making accurate and timely decisions in such complex scenarios while balancing cost considerations and navigating the healthcare system adds to the mental and emotional stress.

The types of contemporary caregiver stress described above amplify the long-standing, outsized **"legacy" stresses and expectations of our profession in society**. We expect, and are expected, to work harder than those in most other kinds of work. We expect to manage with less sleep and still perform with energy, competence, and compassion. We are routinely exposed to some of the most intense of human scenarios and circumstances—blood and guts, observed physical and emotional misery, life-and-death decision making—a consistent exposure to trauma that can have a significant emotional impact on our well-being. We train away much of our early adulthood in an unusual, pressure-packed training culture. This immersion creates a risk of our sacrificing our "well-rounded" individual selves in service of deeper competence in our narrower professional identifications. This sacrifice may leave some of us less self-aware, and as a result inexperienced and vulnerable in other realms of adulthood, including relationships, parenting, fulfillment in activities and interests outside of the workplace, and financial competency.

As is true for our patients, we too can benefit from the use of basic mindfulness tactics to be more adaptive and centered amidst a busy workload. Immersed in the flow of demanding moments at work, many of us wall off or ignore incipient signals of the impact of that stress, pushing on blindly with our tasks until the signals become alarms or worse.

Our well-honed skills in observation of and eliciting signs and symptoms need not be only directed toward our patients. For many healthcare professionals, our own internal experience is an undiscovered country. Earlier identification of and familiarity with our own unique, individual presentations of encroaching stress is an obvious kind of self-diagnostic skill. The intention in early and accurate diagnosis is no different for ourselves than it is for our patients. Regular, even brief practices can reinforce our **increasing self-awareness of tension** and the opportunity to attend to it for our own and our patients' benefit. A regular, repetitive "touching base" with our interior experience in basic meditation reinforces and conditions a state of awareness that rides along with us through our work day, its efforts, interactions, and stresses. We can diagnostically tend simultaneously to others and ourselves. Being more present in each moment, our productivity and efficiency improves, even during busy and demanding times.

As has been described, mindfulness practices not only sharpen our attention and concentration inward and outward—a "diagnostic" benefit—but also help activate the body's relaxation response, reducing the physiological effects of stress. **Mindfulness serves us therapeutically** in this way to feel calmer and more centered amidst a busy workload. We improve not only our perception of but also emotional regulation of our reactivity to the obvious triggers for tension and frustration—including the sheer effort overload, bureaucratic obstacles and burdens, and at times unattainable expectations.

Mindfulness tactics serve us well in attending to and pushing back on the multitude of stressors that can "flood the landscape" of a demanding job. Cultivating reduced reactivity to those stressors clears the field and so reduces wasted energy and effort. That "flood control" also allows for an essential aspect of our work to be attended to with less distraction: **empathy.** We can directly cultivate compassion and empathy as part of our regular mindfulness practices. The increased sense of empathy positively impacts patient care by allowing us to connect more authentically with our patients, understand their needs, and provide more personalized and attentive treatment.

The demands described above are incredibly common in today's medical ecosystem. Of course, the impacts of working harder and faster, being swamped by too much data, and facing the challenge of an ever-increasing learning curve are not unique to healthcare. Other highly technical and complex professions have their own versions, albeit with variations on the "outer" landscape of external professional expectations. To understand our own challenges more fully, it's worthwhile to turn our attention to our "inner" landscape—to look in the mirror, metaphorically.

While each of us have our own unique character, we who choose healthcare as a career commonly identify with some temperamental qualities and aspirations to know better—foremost among them being intellectual gratification, being thought highly of, and compassion for others. These capacities are ideally beneficial to society as well as ourselves as individuals. Yet these same temperamental styles, if we poorly understand how they operate in ourselves personally, can actually cause problems in our work, both in quality and our fulfillment. Next, we'll take a look at that.

The Healthcare Professional's Temperament: Fulfillment and Risk

While each of us is of course distinct individuals, we can nevertheless frame some "archetypa" character styles of healthcare professionals: constellations of psychological attributes drive our work and fulfillment, but which can also pose risks to those ideals [6]. The individual benefits to each of us are manifold and varied but can be categorized into three main aspects of fulfillment that our own temperamental tendencies align with intellect, personal self-respect, and compassion.

These aspirations—smart, well-thought of, and caring—are of course hard to argue with in terms of vectors of life success. Ironically, striving mindlessly for these apex qualities can actually generate problems at work and at home. In "As You Like It," Shakespeare has us consider the risks when one desire(s) too much of a good thing. Taking our cue from the bard, each ideal also can clue us into its associated risks and blind spots in terms of stress and even burnout when we strive for any or all of them mindlessly.

- **Intellectual fulfillment** in medical work stems from the complex and intellectually stimulating nature of the job. Medical professionals engage in a lifelong pursuit of knowledge and continuously challenge ourselves to stay updated with the latest research, advancements, and best practices in the field. We embrace the opportunity to solve intricate diagnostic puzzles, analyze complex medical cases, and develop innovative treatment plans. A wide range of specialties and subspecialties each offer unique and varied challenges and opportunities for our intellectual growth. Our challenge in applying our expertise in critical thinking, problem-solving skills, and evidence-based decision making to contribute to the well-being of patients brings a deep sense of satisfaction.
- An outsized drive toward mastery is a familiar characteristic of many of us in the field. The cognitive abilities required likely self-select for those of us motivated by a heightened need for **perfectionism.** Yet these tendencies can also lead us toward **poor adaptability to the inevitable uncertainties**, ambiguities, and

imperfections of the too-often frail and fragile processes we encounter in health care. Perfectionism may contribute to **excessive self-criticism, fear of making mistakes, and an overwhelming sense of responsibility**, which ironically can hinder effective decision making and increase the likelihood of medical errors. Without some adaptability, we "threatened perfectionists" may defend more actively with a "**fixation on the fix**"—insistent on achieving solutions where there may not be clear ones. We can mindlessly lean on a reflexive overemphasis on tests, procedures, and low-yield treatments.

- **Personal fulfillment** is directly available in our field. It shows in the form of helping others in their time of need. The ability to provide compassionate care, offer comfort and support to patients and their families during challenging circumstances, and witness positive health outcomes can be incredibly rewarding. Our rigorous training and dedication put into building a medical career fosters a valid sense of pride and accomplishment. Achieving professional milestones, receiving recognition from peers, and being respected for one's knowledge and skills contribute to our personal fulfillment. Of course, there is also personal and family financial fulfillment, with those rewards reflecting the significant time, effort, and financial resources invested in our education and training, providing a sense of security and standard of living.
- Yet an exaggerated desire to be thought well of, while more difficult to own up to than perfectionism, can create its own type of suffering when not tempered by mindful self-awareness. In psychoanalytic terms, this narcissistic style—a **hypersensitive need to see oneself as worthy and even extraordinary**—is seen as a defense against an insecure, fragile sense of unconditional, and inherent self-worth. The idealization from our patients that often comes with the white coat, even before any positive outcomes is certainly fulfilling. Yet we can collude on that idealized "construction" of us. If (or perhaps when) that idealization inevitably gets challenged in the setting of poor responses to treatment, or bureaucratic/institutional obstacles and delays, we are often the front-facing target for tension and grievance. Those of us with poor self-awareness of our own **ego-driven blind spots** may respond to this "denting of the self" poorly, whether in a more active way, via confrontation with the patient, or via a more passive response of retreat into inaction.
- **Compassionate fulfillment** adds a profound, though sometimes overlooked dimension to our profession. We witness the resilience and strength of the human spirit in the face of adversity. We attend to patients overcoming immense challenges, experiencing unexpected recoveries. We witness the birth of new life. Such experiences can remind us of the privilege we have to be part of these transformative moments. Compassion is at the core of our work, a driving force. Our opportunity to experience empathy and provide genuine care for others is uncommon in the world of contemporary work. We have the privilege of participating in relationships, every day, that foster trust, dignity, and respect. Alleviating suffering, both physically and emotionally, pays us a dividend beyond the intellectual and personal: a deep sense of fulfillment that transcends the boundaries of medical practice.

We should be aware of the risk of a frankly **counterfeit form of this fulfillment**—**"false altruism"** is a useful term for this risk. Physicians may reflexively, mindlessly extend extra time and effort in professional service in a way that appears as a transcendent opening in compassion to patients' suffering but actually operates as a "masked" form of the narcissistic style noted above. The apparent selflessness in this style can mask an ego-driven **"need to be needed"**; as such, it is sometimes referred to by the psychoanalytic term "counter-dependency." We may avoid and suppress valid frustrations at feeling overburdened and devalued in the job via a costume of giving more and doing more. With little awareness of this style operating in us (and of the tension we are suppressing), we may ignore the imbalances in our broader personal and family lives that are inevitably generated. It threatens a healthier, more balanced direction of personal resources both within and outside our professional role.

Mindfulness practices serve as an incremental way to help us better identify and adapt to the external and internal phenomena in our life experience, both in and away from our rewarding but demanding work. We've addressed the pressures from outside and the tendencies from inside that we're better off not ignoring, but instead being more mindfully aware of. Both understanding the stresses of this current moment in the profession and getting to know our own "mix" of archetypal styles and tendencies can benefit both the professional and the profession—good for us workers, and good for our work.

Prior to finishing this survey of our individual experiences as healthcare professionals and the stresses and impacts thereof, it's important to look directly at the worst-case outcome. The now well-used term "burnout" is not a clinical one but is nevertheless useful in identifying a profession in crisis.

Burnout

The term "burnout" has actually been used for a couple of decades, initially framed by the Texas Medical Association in the 1990s. It is a state of chronic physical, emotional, and mental exhaustion that occurs among us healthcare professionals in response to prolonged and excessive stress.

While the impacts of healthcare stress are indelibly personal, the parallel concern is the risk of erosion of the physician–patient relationship, which has profound implications for our delivery of quality care. We often find ourselves with limited time for each patient due to increasing workloads and administrative burdens.

As a result, our patient encounters may be rushed. Our basic eye contact is impacted as we pivot from screen to patient and back. Our attention is stretched thin, distractibility increased. The opportunity for meaningful interaction and trust-building is threatened, and our alliance and all that goes with it—trust, compliance, effectiveness, and ultimately, outcomes. It is impacting ourselves and our intentions—bad for the workers, and bad for the work.

Besides the risks of medical errors, decreased job satisfaction, and increased risks of substance abuse and mental health issues, burned-out professionals are also more likely to consider leaving the medical profession altogether, leading to a shortage of experienced healthcare professionals.

The Texas Medical Society's initial examination of physician burnout identified these three stages:

- **"Stage 1"** defines the earliest symptoms, framed as the initial effects of "stress arousal"—a mismatch between our "reserve" versus our external expectations of our work. Signs include irritability, anxiety, insomnia, changes in attention, concentration, and distraction. Physical symptoms such as palpitations and increased blood pressure can occur.
- **"Stage 2"** is indicated as the signs in Stage 1 become more persistent, as well as attempts at some compensatory, defensive short-term "fixes." These behaviors include being chronically late to work and in charting; emerging apathy, cynicism, and resentment; increased use of caffeine, alcohol and other mood modifiers; and a drop in social and intimate contacts.
- **"Stage 3"** signals a worsening of the prior signs and behaviors, but especially the onset of a more global exhaustion. We feel drained and depleted with diminishing returns from the "fixes.: Besides physical and cognitive fatigue and impacts on common somatic markers of stress (pain, headache, Gi disturbances), clinical depression is common. Most worrying is the emergence of escape fantasies—from work, friends, family contact, and especially our professional identity. Suicidal ideation and attempts become more likely, especially when social isolation leaves no outlet for support and help.

The cumulative effect of these external factors on burnout is far-reaching and ominous. The healthcare website Medscape's *Physician Depression and Burnout Report 2023* [7], surveying over 9000 physicians across most specialties, found an alarming 53% of physicians reporting that they were burned out. The downstream effects are daunting, with over 120,000 physicians quitting through the end of the COVID era, and around 25% of current physicians considering leaving the profession entirely by 2026.

Most ominous is the rate of suicide, already historically higher in physicians and nurses than in many other professions, and on the rise in the last 5 years [8]. Published data on the topic are generally considered inaccurate, as physician suicide is often underreported, as we and our colleagues often find defining ourselves in this end-game of the "sick-role" a dissonant, unacceptable one. Such is the "secret handshake" of a high-stress profession in minimizing our losses and traumas.

Malpractice and Mindfulness

One of the more stressful moments in a clinical career is "the letter"—notifying a healthcare professional about being sued for medical malpractice. It's an experience that inevitably can elicit a range of intense emotions. Besides its legal and financial implications, malpractice processes can be profoundly troubling psychological events that can impact our wellbeing and our functioning in the midst of the drama.

The stress of malpractice litigation on physicians [9] is a significant and pervasive issue within our profession, with impacts before, during, and after the legal actions occur.

We are entrusted with and accept responsibility for the well-being of our patients. Yet the fear of making a mistake that could lead to a malpractice lawsuit can weigh heavily. The persistent—pressure to provide the best possible care while navigating complex medical situations—especially with the current trends in increasing workloads in clinical and bureaucratic effort—can take a toll on our physical and mental health. The fear of being sued can lead us into the "crouch" of defensive medicine, conditioning us to lean toward excess/unnecessary testing and treatment as a bulwark from the risks of potential legal action. This not only drives up healthcare costs but also detracts from the quality of patient care.

If and when legal action occurs, the legal process surrounding malpractice claims can be protracted and emotionally draining. Depositions, court appearances, and the scrutiny of their medical decisions by legal experts all contribute. The financial burdens can also be substantial, especially for specialists in high-risk fields, further adding to the stress and financial strain. Even if a physician ultimately prevails in a lawsuit, the process can leave lasting emotional scars and erode our confidence in our abilities going forward.

A particular trouble spot for those involved in malpractice legalities emanates from a sound legal recommendation that nevertheless amplifies the emotional stress; "don't talk about it." This "gag order" or confidentiality requirement is often imposed to protect the legal strategy of the healthcare institution or insurance company involved in the case. The isolation that comes with not being able to talk about their experience with colleagues, friends, or even family can lead to feelings of loneliness and helplessness. Sharing experiences and seeking advice from peers who may have gone through similar situations can be a valuable source of comfort and guidance. When physicians are denied this outlet, they may find it more challenging to process their emotions. Professionals may already be dealing with guilt, self-doubt, and anxiety about the patient's outcome. Being unable to share these emotions with trusted individuals can truly exacerbate our distress. It can also create a sense of secrecy and shame, as if there is something to hide, further adding to the emotional burden.

No tactic or practice can eliminate the range of stress-driven states that this process causes. That said, the mindfulness techniques elaborated on above can soften the acute tension, allow for clearer decision making, and especially address the potent struggles with judgment and grievance that are a common aspect of the legal process.

- **Basic breath meditation** is a default recommendation, with its ability to generate momentary calm.
- More advanced tactics can involve "**sitting with" emotional aspects of the situation,** either as they spontaneously flood the mind during meditation, or deliberately "bidden"—with an intention not to head down a "rabbit hole" of rumination, but instead identify the somatic, emotional, and thought aspects of the event in the mind. This practice can help "normalize" the event in terms of softening the sharp anxiety, grievance, and tension, through repetitive review and observation.
- Lastly, working with an aspirational ideal of **compassion**—for the suffering self in a difficult situation primarily, but also for others involved in the drama—can be challenging but effective. Similarly, we can work with the ideal of **gratitude** that naturally exists in self-love and nurture, but also for one's support of others, colleagues, and even for the mindfulness practice itself in helping soothe the tension of the moment.

In these ways and others, incorporating mindfulness practices can help physicians build resilience and emotional intelligence, ultimately mitigating the negative impact of malpractice stress on our mental and emotional well-being.

In Summary: The Mindful Healthcare Professional

What does a "mindful healthcare professional" look like? The risk in this overview is to idealize mindfulness, framing it out as some panacea. We may lionize those who "have it," judging the mindful more positively compared to those who aren't interested. There's irony in such judgment about adherence to a practice that supposedly holds nonjudgment as an aspiration. In any event, it's worthy to reiterate the ideal, and the attributes that cultivating our self-awareness can foster.

The mindful healthcare professional is an individual who practices mindfulness ideally in both our personal and professional lives, incorporating its principles into our approach to patient care and work environment. Such a professional embodies intentions that enhance our ability to provide compassionate, patient-centered care while maintaining our own well-being and fulfillment. Four key intentions highlight this practice:

- **Presence and Awareness:** Mindful healthcare professionals work to be optimally present and attentive during interactions with patients and colleagues. They cultivate awareness of their thoughts, emotions, and bodily sensations, which helps them better understand their patients' needs and respond empathetically.
- **Compassionate, Empathic Care:** Mindful healthcare professionals demonstrate genuine care and compassion for our patients, empathizing with their

struggles, fears, and pain. We encourage a patient-centered approach, considering the patient's unique needs, preferences, and values without judgment, and promoting open dialogue and collaborative decision making.
- **Emotional Regulation:** Mindfulness helps healthcare professionals manage our emotions effectively, preventing burnout and compassion fatigue. We can identify and acknowledge our feelings without judgment becoming overwhelmed, enabling us to maintain composure during challenging situations.
- **Resilience:** Mindful healthcare professionals use mindfulness practices for our own benefit in building resilience, helping us to bounce back from difficult experiences and maintain a positive outlook. We recognize that mindfulness practices benefit us personally, help us approach work with optimal focus, and allow us to model resilience in our patients and colleagues.

The specifics of how we can engage mindfulness tactics are, of course, really no different from the range of options we can provide to our patients. As was described in more detail in Chap. 3, our options include seeking out **direct, in-person** provider teaching whether in an individual or group setting; individual practice using **printed, digital, audio/podcast, video, and/or smartphone app resources** for learning introductory basic meditation and other mindful practices. As with any other individual, any of us may gravitate toward particular kinds of routes; some may find the stillness of sitting difficult and find mindful movement practices like yoga, Qi Gong, or Tai Chi more accessible and effective in sharpening awareness and reducing tension. More open-ended work toward personal or spiritual/contemplative experience may attract some; for others, our own use of the brief "core four" tactics featured in Chap. 4 (breath awareness, scanning, visualization, and gratitude/compassion) is sufficient to help manage our own work and personal stresses.

A couple of final comments on launching and then sticking with these practices are in order. First, healthcare professionals can be a famously impatient lot, borne of adaptation to the expectations on outcomes and efficiency. The initial patience involved with sitting in patient (often painful) observation of experience, whether of a simple breath or of our entire landscape of mind in the moment, can be difficult at first; the judgments ("a waste of time!" "New Age hokum!" "nothing's happening!" "everything's happening!") can and will fly. As we would advise any patient, we can take the advice ourselves to give our own initial practice some intention, time (4 weeks is a good initial interval), and effort, without a quick hook for some early struggle or disappointment.

Also, it's better to make our initial foray into practice a standard rather than PRN event. If all we have predictably is 5 min on rising, then that's what we got—schedule it. It can be helpful to also consider introducing a brief "core four" tactic, tied not to a scheduled time, but an event. A brief sitting with compassion and gratitude a few minutes before a morning bloc of office visits can set a tone for that type of work. A quick scan just before scrubbing in helps tighten awareness and perhaps loosen some physical tension. A quiet moment of breathing practice after a code in the ER can truly help us decompress from that intensity.

It also can't be stressed enough how keeping notes throughout the process can assist the practitioner to hone in on and improve the specific weaknesses of our practices, just as ongoing vitals, ins and outs, and laboratory studies allow us to do for our patients and their disease. While many smartphone apps allow for keeping metrics of our time devoted to meditation, personal journaling, digitally or by pen, our subjective experiences can be an invaluable addition to the process. The same can be said for a friend, loved one, or even a team of individuals who partake in the practice alongside us and are available for mutual/shared contemplative exploration.

Developing mindfulness through practice creates a capacity for adaptation, emotional regulation, and ready access to empathy; that capacity remains available for our use, all life long. While individuals benefit each in our own unique ways, mindfulness can generate a powerful, "viral" effect on others through modeling. Physicians and other healthcare professionals inevitably act as role models for our peers and colleagues, for good or not; such is the responsibility of our role. Mindful professionals foster compassion, inspire mutual responsibility, and create a ripple effect that motivates team members to create a culture of transparency and honesty. Next, we will explore how to cultivate a mindful medical workplace.

Key Points
- Mindful healthcare professionals can incorporate mindfulness principles into both personal and professional life, can intentionally prioritize presence and awareness during interactions, demonstrate compassion and empathy, manage emotions effectively, and build resilience to provide patient-centered care while maintaining personal well-being.
- Healthcare professionals can engage in mindfulness practices through various methods, including in-person teaching, individual practice, mindful movement, and the "core four" tactics.
- Initiating mindfulness practice may require patience and consistency, with an initial commitment of at least 4 weeks to allow time for adjustment. Keeping notes and journaling can assist in tracking progress, weaknesses, and subjective experiences in mindfulness practice.
- Role Modeling: Mindful healthcare professionals serve as role models, inspiring compassion, transparency, and a culture of honesty among colleagues, ultimately benefiting the healthcare workplace.
- Overall, mindfulness is seen as a valuable tool for healthcare professionals to address burnout, cope with stress, and enhance the quality of patient care while preserving their own well-being.

References

1. Rink LC, Oyesanya TO, Adair KC, Humphreys JC, Silva SG, Sexton JB. Stressors among healthcare workers: a summative content analysis. Glob Qual Nurs Res. 2023;10:23333936231161127. https://doi.org/10.1177/23333936231161127. PMID: 37020708; PMCID: PMC10068501

References

2. Gunja MZ, et al. Stressed out and burned out: the global primary care crisis—findings from the 2022 international health policy survey of primary care physicians (Commonwealth Fund, Nov. 2022).
3. Schäfer WLA, van den Berg MJ, Groenewegen PP. The association between the workload of general practitioners and patient experiences with care: results of a cross-sectional study in 33 countries. Hum Resour Health. 2020;18(1):76. https://doi.org/10.1186/s12960-020-00520-9. PMID: 33066776; PMCID: PMC7565810
4. How administrative burdens can harm health. Health Affairs Health Policy Brief, October 2, 2020. https://doi.org/10.1377/hpb20200904.405159.
5. Docs Struggle to Keep Up With the Flood of New Medical Knowledge. Here's Advice—Medscape—Mar 02, 2023.
6. Sazima G. The hateful patient revisited: a transactional view of difficult physician-patient relationships. Psychiat Times. 2015;32(6)
7. Kane L. "I cry but no one cares": physician burnout & depression report 2023. Medscapecom. 2023. www.medscape.com/slideshow/2023-lifestyle-burnout-6016058#2.
8. Gold KJ, Schwenk TL, Sen A. Physician suicide in the United States: updated estimates from the national violent death reporting system. Psychol Health Med. 2021;27(7):1563–75.
9. Charles SC, Wilbert JR, Franke KJ. Sued and non-sued physicians' self-reported reactions to malpractice litigation. Am J Psychiatry. 1985;142(4):437–40.

Chapter 7
Mindfulness in Healthcare Teams

In this survey of the uses and benefits of mindfulness throughout the healthcare landscape, we've moved in this section from a patient-centered focus to attend to us caregivers. To fully explore how mindfulness skills may impact and benefit us, in the last chapter, we focused on individuals—physicians, nurses, and other healthcare professionals—and our particular aspirations and stressors.

We open out now to a broader landscape: how we interact and collaborate as teams, from the familiar MD/RN relationship in any routine office visit to more complex systems of whole clinics, hospitals, and health systems. We'll complete this "field trip" of the healthcare ecosystem with a chapter devoted to integrating mindfulness into our various training programs, so that the capacity of mindfulness can be of the broadest benefit, built into the training experience. From the outset of our professional lives, mindfulness training can help us incentivize healthy emotional development professionally and personally and reinforce our core intention in providing competent and compassionate care.

In this chapter, we'll explore:

The **current landscape of healthcare teams** (office teams, clinics, and systems) and their challenges, in terms of both external and internal stressors

- The impacts of healthcare workplace stress on **teams (competence, communication, and care)** and the worsening concerns about **"team burnout."**
- How **mindfulness practices can make a difference** on larger scales from teams to larger systems.
- Some considerations and concrete tactics in **implementing the "mindful healthcare workplace."**

Those Were the Days

Some of us in the healthcare ecosystem, especially those of us longer in the tooth, can summon a sense of nostalgia and wistfulness for the "old days" of medicine. A single physician handling most aspects of patient care ourselves, from offering an empathic ear to diagnosing ailments and prescribing remedies, was the bygone, sepia-toned norm.

The impacts of exploding medical knowledge, technological complexity, and the inevitability of corporate/profit-based pressures have had a profound impact on contemporary medical care. With these trends, it has become increasingly challenging for individual physicians to practice in the "legacy" standard triad (MD, RN, and office manager). While the core capacities of compassionate care and technical competence continue as essentials, medical practice has undergone a significant transformation, shifting in many if not most settings from individual MDs to collaborative medical teams.

Today's medical office bustles with multiple doctors, nurses, other valuable practitioners such as Physician Assistants and Nurse Practitioners, and office staff. That office is often part of a larger care system with its own byzantine referral patterns, as well as insurance-based directives and restrictions. Once a metaphorical community of "family farms," the healthcare landscape more and more trends toward a few "Con-Agras" [1]—larger systems with increasing emphasis (and resulting pressures) on standardization and productivity.

Our workplaces are morphing to meet these changing needs and expectations, aiming for accuracy and productivity while sustaining the fragile but essential trust and alliance with our patients. Today's optimal medical workplace can be a busy but focused, fulfilling team effort. It can also be a breeding ground for psychological stress and conflict. The sheer volume of patients, the complexity of medical cases, and the pressure to deliver high-quality care within limited time frames can take a toll on the mental well-being of healthcare professionals. Where medical teams composed of specialists from different disciplines have emerged, a more comprehensive and multidisciplinary approach to patient care can follow but also a clash of processes, styles, and expectations.

Failure to address the current stresses on healthcare teams and systems can lead to a cascade of detrimental outcomes;

- A **lack of attentional focus**, stemming from limited self-awareness, can hinder our effective decision making in both routine and critical situations.
- The absence of mindfulness practices can exacerbate **communication breakdowns** among team members, leading to misunderstandings and medical errors that compromise patient safety.
- The absence of mindfulness-based coping mechanisms to cultivate emotional regulation could leave healthcare professionals **ill-equipped to process the emotional toll of our work, potentially leading to compassion fatigue** and decreased empathy toward our patients.

- Healthcare teams, like with individuals, can become overwhelmed by mounting stress, resulting in higher levels of **burnout and decreased job satisfaction and retention**.
- Inadequate attention to mindfulness might **further erode work–life balance**, exacerbating the physical and mental health challenges faced by healthcare workers.

As with individuals, healthcare teams can leverage mindfulness practices for the good of the work—improved communication, interaction, and care. Mindfulness is also for the good of the workplace. "Mindful" teams can operate with a more unified, reinforced intention of competent, compassionate care; getting along better with our colleagues; and can forgive the inevitable conflicts and tensions that arise with less distress and drama. Fulfillment in teamwork can become contagious and reinforcing.

As with our survey of the current moment for individual healthcare pros, we can extrapolate some similar trends and stresses to care teams and systems.

Healthcare Teams and Stress

We've identified three powerful trends in the healthcare ecosystem that impact individual productivity versus overwhelm, and fulfillment versus stress-driven burnout. Just as they do on individual caregivers' attitudes and performance, those pressures also resonate in a team setting in terms of tone and behavior, and can commonly affect the rest of the team and setting.

The **workload and productivity pressures** that we identified as a potent challenge for individual healthcare professionals also impact our functioning in teams. Team healthcare operates best as a collaborative effort, working together to provide comprehensive care. When roles become blurred due to increased pressure and expectations, it can lead to conflicts and misunderstandings among team members about who is responsible for what aspect of patient care.

An ancillary concern to our shared management of this complexity is what can be termed the "front facing" effect on interactions with our patients and colleagues. Our patients, often carrying the tension of uncertainty about new or worsening medical illness, now must inevitably have many more discrete interactions with multiple individuals in our teams and systems than ever before. These interactions include scheduling, payment and insurance issues, receiving clinical/lab information, and fielding patients' questions, anxieties, and complaints. This increasing complexity in care requires greater precision in our interactions and communications. In attending to the stress this places on patients, predictably clear, consistent, and empathic communications from any and all of the healthcare team involved are truly important. Yet those expectations are more difficult to entrain and sustain in a team than via an individual caregiver.

Affiliate/allied providers of care may be working with more patients and with less familiarity, and even being tasked with taking on responsibilities that may extend beyond one's traditional scope of practice—raising more stress about ethics and liability in the service of output. Secondary pressures about the limits of work expectations can involve fears of letting down the team in terms of effort, commitment, and capability.

Bureaucratic and administrative burdens, including tending to the leviathan of today's electronic health record (EHR) expectations, are essential but at times confounding in coordinating contemporary team-based care. More patience than ever is required with bureaucratic obstacles being a shared team task.

While teams can provide complementary and mutually informed perspectives to improve diagnosis and treatment planning, multiple professionals documenting each of our own contributions can cause a flood of information through the EHR. For some professionals, pasting and copying all past notes for completeness and/or a sense of legal obligation has generated a flood of repetitive information. The result is not necessarily of "more is better," but instead of a morass of data for clinicians to cull through. Clinical leaders and allied staff alike can be weighed down by IT systems that add unpredictability, require a daunting learning curve for initial facility with use, and frequent retraining on new, changed features in keeping and conveying clinical information. Bureaucratic and administrative burdens can and often must be offloaded or spread out, to fairly and equitably participate in the extra effort required. But that aspiration also requires a team that shares that sense of a mutual, equitable vision.

Having everyone all perfectly "singing the same tune" in terms of patient interaction is, of course, unrealistic. But broad variations in how multiple professionals interact with patients in a pressurized work setting can generate a perception of the whole team, office, and even care systems as compassion-challenged, and even incompetent or uncaring. A frazzled, tense work setting can leak out into unempathic interactions with patients and staff, and result in patient frustration, complaints, and even social media "doxxing." [2] Hard-won reputations for **compassionate care** can erode quickly in this way.

While any group of people in a difficult, shared task can ally or scrum based on the circumstances, it makes good sense that mindfulness practices can help here in both preemptive and reactive ways. The mutual affiliation among team members with shared roots in mindful self-awareness in a basic sense means they just get along better. We are more likely to directly address and work through interpersonal problems that can arise. The core "outlook" inherent in mindfulness work, grounded in our shared human experience of being imperfect, cultivates interactions that emphasize being compassionate and accepting over judgmental and poorly adaptive. Organizations that can embrace the underlying tenets of mindfulness—cultivation of better awareness of self and others to enhance clinical competence, communication, compassion, and self-care—can see those tenets reflected in patient trust and appreciation, even within a team approach.

Mindfulness and Healthcare Team Dynamics

Besides exploring the external stresses acting on healthcare teams, we may also look "inward," at psychological team dynamics. This spans the broader issue of the team's overall mission/vision, to the day-to-day, moment-to-moment interactions that can benefit from mindfulness-aided insight. Improved individual self-awareness can become improved team awareness and collaboration. Or not.

In the last chapter, we framed out some "archetypal" character styles and aspirations of individual healthcare professionals: intellect, personal self-respect, and compassion. These personal aspirations—smart, well-thought of, and caring—of course also can manifest as holistic team goals. Teams, regardless of size and reach, are ultimately made up of individuals contracting with each other for those shared intentions. The broader reputational goals of an office, clinic, or system should align with our individual reputations for clinical competence, effective communication, and a foundation of compassion.

The issues/dynamics/adaptability of each person involved inevitably have at least some impacts on the quality of the collaboration. This impacts clinical outcomes, as well as the fulfillment of and stress on fellow collaborators. While "one bad apple" may rarely take down the whole enterprise, individual states of self-awareness matter, with consequences for the health and stability of the team and the enterprise. This reality raises the ante on making a concerted effort for full buy-in of all, and to making mindfulness training available to all, throughout the team, clinic, and system.

We can extrapolate our individual temperamental archetypes to how they manifest in a team setting:

- **Clinical competence** in medical teams ideally is an aspiration that germinates from the traits of the individuals on the team: a love of knowledge, solving problems, and mastery. This shared intention has its own momentum when embraced and cultivated in a team setting. At best, it demonstrates a positive attitude among effective teams both in expectations of high-level service provision. Sustaining that competence requires investing in time and resources for team members to collaborate and mutually support each other. Team members ideally can complement each other's strengths and compensate for weaknesses.

- When individual healthcare providers with strong intellectual competence collaborate effectively, they can contribute to better patient outcomes. When workplace stress is not identified and attended to, individual competence can be nullified by communication breakdowns and downfield impacts in care provision. Our individual drives toward perfection can generate frustration as "our team" struggles. Interpersonal conflicts, reduced collaboration and cohesion, and fingerprinting can result and further erode a shared sense of pride and belonging in the healthcare team. Burnout and staff turnover only accelerate the loss of cohesion and a shared mission of team competence.

- Healthcare professionals' desires toward **being valued and respected** ideally fuels a workplace-wide mission to reflect that in attention to team unity and cohesion. We can model our self-respect in how we treat our colleagues, mirroring that behavior in patient interactions. Poor individual self-awareness fuels a different outcome in terms of team behaviors. Respect for the setting, the institution, and even our profession as a whole, is a quality that can erode in the midst of unattended-to stress. As workplace tension escalates and a sense of mutual respect dwindles, lowered expectations for the team can become normalized. Ultimately, both team members and our patients suffer.
- Our temperamental tendency toward work that emanates from **empathy and compassion** can scale to the healthcare team as a potent, shared sense of kindness in care that can be deeply motivating, even a reason why many professionals prefer working in teams to individual practice. At least, individuals in healthcare teams can help each other buffer the stresses of the work to resist "compassion fatigue." At best, as teams, we can reinforce and amplify the fulfillment of being of service.

However, workplace stress can erode team dynamics. Empathy as a shared team aspiration can fall prey to individual conflicts and resentments. Colleagues who are "behind the curve" in terms of our own mindfulness, our own "blind spots" thereof, often can remain less tuned in and empathic, leaving office staff as a (or "the") buffer to soothe patients and salvage questionable "bedside manner." Teams often shoulder the emotional burden of patient stress, as patients may not feel comfortable opening up to certain physicians. The values of both that buffer against burnout and the shared pride in a compassionate workplace can wither. That shift may not become obvious to ourselves and our peers until it is already so to patients and referral sources.

The emotional stress of teams, as with individuals, is amplified by the gross increase in clinical complexity, market-based pressures, and distractions that serve to erode our empathic, compassionate approach to others in suffering. The dreaded "burnout" that external stressors visit on individual caregivers can extend to the ecosystem itself.

What Could Happen? Team Burnout

Stress in healthcare team settings can manifest in various ways due to the demanding nature of the work, the high stakes involved, and the complex interactions between team members. With increasing clinical complexity, in addition to insurance and administrative tensions, "burnout" can extend to all in the ecosystem.

What if we ignore the warning signs? Just keep our heads down and push harder? We can use the Chap. 5 framework of the phases of individual burnout and apply them to team/interactive settings:

- **"Stage 1":** This initial stress "arousal" phase reflects a growing gap between teams' capabilities and advancing work demands. While individual team members may manifest this in our own shifts (irritability, anxiety, insomnia, distraction, and somatic stress symptoms), group effects include:

- Breakdowns in effective communication, which impact on clinical decision making and medical errors
- Decreased cohesion, with an increase in minor interpersonal conflicts, and downfield effects of reduced mutual trust, and more team members then "going solo" rather than collaboration in decision making
- Signs of diminished job satisfaction, fulfillment, and enthusiasm among team members

- **"Stage 2":** As with individual burnout, the signs of team burnout become more persistent but may be variable as each individual responds with their own adaptability or lack thereof to the stress of the work setting. These include:
  - More frequent breakdowns in communication and secondary grievance and tension that colors subsequent interactions.
  - Worsening workplace cohesion, with "not getting along" becoming more the norm than the outlier; teams may often split into factions based on persistent conflicts, judgments, and blame, as well as tension among team leaders.
  - Worsening job productivity and satisfaction, including delays/gaps in non-clinical tasks (charting, scheduling, office upkeep, and protocol); an increase in medical leaves of absence due to stress, absenteeism, signs of "escape"/lost team talent due to the erosive workplace setting.

- **"Stage 3":** A progression of the prior signs and behaviors occurs in individuals and also in teams; the settling in of a more global sense of burnout become the norm:
  - Frequent communication conflicts and information exchange generate more frequent clinical mistakes and second guessing among team members.
  - Helplessness in any changing of the dysfunction can lead to a resultant retreat of individuals from a "team first" to survival mode, "take care of myself" attitudes, resistance to adopting new practices and procedures.
  - A palpable drop in empathy in clinical interactions, with "compassion fatigue" a manifestation of the loss of team values
  - High turnover rates occur with consistent departure of team members due to burnout and dissatisfaction (Table 7.1).

We can stick with the current burnout-leaning trends and hope for the best. We can try to manage and tolerate a sense of increasing grief and grievance for a profession falling further from our patients and our own idealized expectations. Much of what ails the current system requires complex structural changes. Yet a more accessible, quick-return effort to implement mindfulness practices in our teams and systems can indeed serve as a foundational and essential interior quality for grappling with today's pressures. The mindful healthcare team is a force multiplier for better care and professional fulfillment. We can speculate on what that would look like.

Table 7.1 Stages of team burnout

Stage 1—Initial stress arousal	Stage 2—Persistent stress response	Stage 3—Global burnout
• Symptoms: Increased individual stress markers (irritability, anxiety), breakdowns in team communication • Effects on Team: Reduced cohesion, minor interpersonal conflicts, diminished job satisfaction • Mindful Intervention: Regular team mindfulness sessions to enhance communication and stress management	• Symptoms: Worsening communication breakdowns, faction formation, increased absenteeism • Effects on Team: Decreased productivity, rising grievances, medical leaves due to stress • Mindful Intervention: Mindfulness-based conflict resolution training and stress-reduction workshops	• Symptoms: Frequent clinical mistakes, loss of team values, high turnover rates • Effects on Team: A pervasive sense of helplessness, retreat into individual survival mode, compassion fatigue • Mindful Intervention: Comprehensive team-building retreats focusing on mindfulness, empathy, and resilience training

Navigating through burnout with mindfulness	The mindful healthcare team—a vision
• Preventative approach: Regular mindfulness practices embedded in team routines to maintain a balanced perspective and mitigate the onset of burnout • Resilience building: Cultivating a team culture of mindfulness to enhance empathy and reduce compassion fatigue • Communication enhancement: Utilizing mindfulness to improve team communication, prevent misunderstandings, and strengthen team cohesion • Addressing systemic issues: While structural changes are complex, mindfulness offers a foundational approach to improve team dynamics and job satisfaction	• Empowered teams: Mindful practices enabling teams to navigate high-pressure environments with clarity and empathy • Patient-centered care: Enhanced focus on patient care through improved team dynamics and reduced burnout • Professional fulfillment: Cultivating a work environment where team members find value and satisfaction in their roles

Team... Mindfulness

In a shared advocacy for positive change, for "re-humanizing" the practice of medicine, there are many moving parts to attend to, beyond the scope of this book. Furthermore, it would be grandiose to propose an institutional commitment to mindfulness as some simplistic "cure" for a complex problem. But apart from any other systemic changes and innovations to be considered, the most cost-effective, low-risk intervention we can make is in our own self-awareness, attention, and ultimately well-being. As with individuals engaging in mindfulness practices to cultivate our own interior understanding of our personal goals, reactions, and blindspots, we can also improve our understanding and management of workplace interactions.

Mindfulness training can foster a re-humanizing of medical team practice; as noted, it's good for the work and good for the workplace. Here are some of the ways we can benefit:

- Basic **flexibility/adaptability of attention improves**, affording greater clarity of decision making and communication.
- Relationships among caregivers have their own dynamics and fulfillments to identify and be more aware of in the work setting. Team members cultivate **a better "reading of the room"** in the daily workplace—identifying familiar temperamental patterning of both ourselves and other team members.
- Mindfulness entrains calmer, **more deliberate responses to angry or conflictual inputs**, both from patients and among staff.
- Better-self-awareness of momentary tensions and judgments leads to less likelihood of those distractors intruding on good care collaboration. When we and our peers are in momentary distress and/or grievance, any of us are prone to "leaking" out that tension: displacing it on others, picking tussles, and other defensive but provocative moves. As individual emotional tensions and conflicts are better identified, **we can operate with less "acting-out"**—employing inappropriate behaviors that are driven often by subconscious or hard-to-hold interior upset.

An associated psychological term that is now part of the social zeitgeist, "**passive-aggressive**," referring to a way of expressing negative emotions, frustration, or resistance indirectly, rather than openly addressing the issues at hand. It's a common workplace contaminant that better team awareness can help reduce. Healthy, open interactions in both language and behavior become the precedent and the expectation.

- Mindfulness-informed teams often generate a sustained, cultivated shared sense about the state of the team in the moment and ongoing expectations for mindful care among all team members. "**Mindful" can be a driving ID** of the clinic, team, and system.
- Mindful team training is **an effective component of onboarding and integrating new staff** into existing teams, reinforcing a team ethos of mutual health and care alongside position-based skills training.

The Mindful Healthcare System

Pulling the focus back even more wide-angled, to larger healthcare systems, the implications of stress on individuals and teams can be seen as wear and tear affecting the cells of a much larger organism. Comparable to the recent pandemic, stress in healthcare systems is a metaphorical virus that may or may not show up as an abrupt, obvious, critical disease state. Yet that wear and tear can simmer silently, if temporarily, in larger systems. A small subset of burned-out professionals or a couple of dysfunctional departments may not trigger immediate attention to the problem in the way stress manifests in smaller teams and settings.

But ignoring the stress weakens large healthcare systems in far-reaching, hard-to-reverse ways, manifesting at various levels within a healthcare organization. Both patients and care providers are affected, and ultimately the quality of care and overall system performance is as well.

As we've reiterated, stressed and less adaptive healthcare providers have reduced time and energy to attention, communication, and empathy. The diminished quality of care breeds patient dissatisfaction and may even deter our patients from seeking necessary medical care or following treatment plans, potentially worsening health outcomes.

Some more tuned-in healthcare systems are monitoring this issue through data collection and analysis, using contemporaneous and sequential surveying of patient and provider input. Larger systems may only become aware of festering trends in these after-the-fact surveys, and via parallel data on absenteeism, decreased productivity, and higher staff turnover.

One particular factor is salient in the diagnostic/monitoring efforts of larger systems, as it is for individuals: minimization of stress as another temperamental quality of us in the profession. The special kind of peer pressure to be iron-clad and stress-proof, inculcated in us from early in training, still operates. As physicians and other professionals have hit and blown past limits of physical and psychological endurance, we are nevertheless rigid in minimizing the negative impacts on us, and may under-report stressful impacts. Systems and individuals can collude in a distorted sense that all's well in this way.

This baked-in, temperamental "stiff upper lip" style has been embedded in our profession for many decades, driven by an existential contract that exchanged outsized expectations of healthcare professionals in terms of effort and endurance for our elevated social and economic position. It took a highly publicized tragedy, the "Libby Zion" case [3], to shine a light on the emotional toll that such demanding work schedules take on physicians. Ms. Zion was a college freshman with depression, admitted to a New York hospital in March 1984 for observation of flu-like symptoms and agitation. She died due to a lethal drug–drug interaction and other management decisions that raised issues about the impact of trainee work schedules, which commonly approached 100 h per week and 36 h per shift. The controversial case had a profound impact on the identification of stress on physician trainees—severe fatigue, sleep deprivation, and impaired decision making, ultimately compromising patient safety.

That tragedy has served as a catalyst for the incremental recognition of the issue of stress, fatigue, and burnout among physicians, especially trainees. It has led to regulatory changes aimed at improving working conditions, reducing errors, and enhancing patient safety, mostly around mandated limits in hours and shifts, less so on the individual and group psychological aspects of practice that mindfulness can be complementary in addressing. Meanwhile, in the almost 40 years since that tragic but influential inflection point for attending to the medical workforce, the work environment has only become more intense for professionals in most cases.

As explored earlier, with building self-awareness through mindfulness training comes greater sensitivity to our interior states—in this case, simmering burnout. HR initiatives toward stress management including mindfulness training, are not generally a costly line item. Yet they are ironically (and often) the first cuts made when systemic failures impacted by stress lead to financial strains on the system. The pricier bill for recruitment and training of replacement staff can lead to a vicious cycle in terms of further talent retention and quality losses.

In addition to the risks of individual and team burnout, an overall erosion of system morale is likely when healthcare workers feel that what and how we do matters less and less in systems tone-deaf to the wellbeing of patients and providers. As more healthcare systems and practices are purchased and managed by far-away entities such as private equity funds, the workers at all levels face increasing pressure for productivity with fewer resources. The human face of medicine may be devalued insidiously but inevitably when the compassionate core of our profession is not attended to.

Mindful healthcare teams reinforce its constituent members in modeling health, fostering compassion, and having the courage to challenge team/system principles when necessary. We inspire each other to take more responsibility and create a ripple effect that can motivate team members to initiate further innovations and healthy change. We work to create a culture of transparency and understanding. These qualities are timeless in healthy human interaction. They have also gained unprecedented prominence in recent times as key features of diversity, equity, and inclusion (DEI) efforts to foster a more inclusive and equitable society. Mindfulness training is an effective tool here, perhaps even a preferable one.

Mindfulness and DEI

DEI (diversity, equity, and inclusion) efforts and initiatives have gained momentum as our society has wrestled with evidence of persistent inequalities and systemic biases that have disadvantaged marginalized groups, and tussled further over responses and solutions.

In the context of healthcare, DEI efforts [4] are aimed at cultivating changes in a healthcare system to value and embrace diversity, ensure equitable access to care, and foster an inclusive environment for patients, healthcare providers, and staff. DEI in medicine recognizes that individuals from various backgrounds, identities, and experiences should receive fair and culturally sensitive treatment, as well as have the opportunity to contribute to and participate in the healthcare field.

Hierarchies—structured/ranked groups based on some judgment of value—are inevitable in any workplace, and not necessarily unfairly discriminatory. Valid ones are based in responsibility, skill level and licensure, age, and experience. There are hierarchies that are less so—gender, race, and sexual orientation are the most obvious ones. Hierarchies can sometimes swamp the reality outside of those rankings—of unconditional respect of others in our work and personal lives, regardless of hierarchy.

In terms of consciousness, a bias refers to a "systematic and often unconscious inclination or predisposition." Explicit biases—overt, even endorsed (if grossly misinformed) inclinations about values or capabilities—are more obvious than ever in workplaces that have become more diverse over time, but still may operate in plain view. Implicit biases are trickier for us to engage, sometimes even more threatening for some to self-reflect on. It's an often reflexive, "mindless" mental shortcut, a part of human cognition that can help us process vast amounts of information quickly, if not accurately. Biases become problematic when they lead to unfair treatment, discrimination, or perpetuation of unequal power dynamics.

The aspiration for individuals to better identify and appreciate the reality of systemic unfairness that some of us have been and continue to be burdened with would seem a sincere, even unarguable one. Nevertheless, organized diversity/equity/inclusion (DEI) programs have, like with so many contemporary social issues, become hyper-politicized. Individual reactions to this effort are varied and have been stoked by a polarizing media landscape into more heat than light, with mindless grievance and locked-in positions as likely as mindful examination of ourselves and our teams.

This political melodrama may lead some to minimize to ignore systemic inequity and bias on one end of the spectrum, perpetuating a persistent social problem. It may lead others with positive intentions in raising awareness to over-dramatize and personalize judgments about others, a prosecutorial approach that rarely persuades individuals toward self-reflection. Proposals and programs, and then backlash, are the order of the moment politically and socially.

Political attempts to delegitimize or even erase the topic aside, greater societal awareness of systemic bias is "out of the bottle." Indeed the backlash is a familiar phenomenon as a societal change is more broadly and consciously opened to. Yet the aspirations of medicine and DEI are both rooted in the shared commitment to fostering an environment where every individual is treated with dignity and respect. The intentions of the DEI project seamlessly align with the goals of the healthcare community, as we both strive to ensure equitable, inclusive access to quality care. The healthcare community holds a unique and influential position in society to actively cultivate (DEI) values and practices. As a field dedicated to promoting well-being, treating illness, and improving quality of life, we healthcare professionals have the capacity to set an example and drive positive change toward a more inclusive and equitable society.

If we take down the intention of DEI work (or of any social movement to raise awareness) to its "studs," it is to effect change in an individual's mental outlook - in this case, to raise awareness of long-standing and persistent structural inequalities, biases, and discriminatory practices that have marginalized some of us based on our race, gender, ethnicity, sexual orientation, and/or socioeconomic status. That aim to enlighten, to change minds, is foundational to a broader goal of translating that awareness into creating systemic and cultural shifts that promote diversity, equity, and inclusion on a broader scale. The intention is rooted in individual awareness—the capacity that mindfulness practices cultivate. The impact of that individual work on a team can be formal, in terms of sustained efforts for programming; but is most potent in reflecting in the everyday actions and interactions of us in manifesting equity and inclusion in our daily work.

Mindfulness, in the context of DEI programming, can—and may need to—play a significant role in achieving these intentions [5]. We can think of using meditation as a "self-study" course—our own interior DEI CME! —to examine our emotions and reactions as they arise naturally. We may even examine them in a systematic way in meditation.

When integrated into DEI efforts [6], mindfulness enhances the effectiveness and depth of the initiatives in these ways:

Self-awareness and Self-reflection: Most importantly, mindfulness encourages individuals to become more attuned to their biases, beliefs, and attitudes. This self-awareness is crucial in better recognizing any unconscious biases that might influence decision making, behavior, and interactions. With a greater self-awareness of our bias-driven "blind spots" and how they operate in our daily judgments and interactions, we can take steps to mitigate their impact and make more equitable choices.

Empathy and Perspective-taking: Mindfulness promotes empathy and compassion by encouraging people to listen actively, suspend judgment, and truly understand others' experiences and perspectives. Mindfulness training, when focused on contemplation of one's poorly recognized implicit beliefs, shines light on them and allows for more deliberate analysis of sometimes long-held perspectives worth re-assessment. Outmoded perspectives no longer operate as potently; dismantling them affords an easier route to empathy for our patients and others with less implicit judgment. This is an essential intention in DEI programming, as it enables individuals to bridge gaps in understanding and recognizing the challenges faced by marginalized groups.

Reducing Reactivity and Conflict: Mindfulness practices help us manage our own emotional reactions, reducing the potential for defensive or confrontational responses. The effect is to manage conflict in a nonaggressive and respectful manner. This creates a safer space for open dialogue and allows participants to engage in constructive conversations about sensitive topics. This is particularly (and ironically!) important for addressing disagreements and misunderstandings that may arise when discussing the complex and sensitive topics of bias itself.

Creating and Sustaining Inclusive Spaces and Attitudes: Mindfulness practices foster a sense of presence and connection, which can be harnessed to create inclusive environments. When individuals are fully present and engaged, they are more likely to make others feel valued and heard, contributing to an inclusive atmosphere. DEI efforts can be emotionally challenging and mentally taxing, given the complex and often emotional nature of the work. Mindfulness practices provide tools for managing stress, avoiding burnout, and maintaining a long-term commitment to inclusivity and fairness.

Better management of grievance, including as it pertains to valid issues of unfair/inequitable treatment in some workplaces, allows for more deliberate than impulsive/reactive responses to that tension. More productive, rather than defensive, responses pave the way for healthier dispute resolution and more importantly, better awareness and sensitivity to equity issues (Table 7.2).

Table 7.2 Mindful DEI in healthcare

Understanding DEI in healthcare:	• **DEI goals:** Aligned with Healthcare: Emphasizes **equal and sensitive treatment for diverse groups**, ensuring fair participation in healthcare roles • **Hierarchies and biases:** Recognizes the existence of structured hierarchies based on skill and responsibility, while **addressing biases based on gender, race, sexual orientation, etc.** • **Challenges of DEI efforts:** Acknowledges the **complexity of societal bias and the controversy surrounding DEI initiatives**
The role of mindfulness in enhancing DEI	• **Promoting self-awareness:** Encourages individuals to recognize and manage unconscious biases, fostering equitable decisions • **Empathy and perspective-taking:** Deepens understanding of others' experiences, bridging gaps and fostering inclusivity • **Reducing reactivity in sensitive conversations:** Empowers calm, respectful engagement in DEI discussions, promoting constructive dialogues • **Sustaining inclusive environments:** Mindfulness enhances the sense of connection and inclusivity in healthcare settings
Practical integration of mindfulness in DEI initiatives	• **Education and training in mindfulness**: Introduce mindfulness practice prior to engaging in DEI discussions or workshops to add onto system-wide DEI meetings • **Creating mindful environments:** Design spaces and culture that encourage mindfulness as part of daily routines • **Leadership embracing mindfulness**: Encourage leaders to model mindful behavior, fostering a culture of mindfulness • **Mindfulness in patient interactions**: Apply mindfulness in patient care to enhance communication and empathy • **Regular mindfulness practice:** Advocate for routine mindfulness practice among staff for firsthand benefits
Implementation strategies for mindful DEI	• **Holistic approach**: Combine education, environment, leadership, and patient care integration for effective mindfulness implementation • **Mindful leadership and champions**: Identify and empower leaders and champions in different healthcare groups and across multiple levels of training and expertise to promote mindfulness • **Group sessions and workshops:** Organize group mindfulness sessions and workshops for staff and patients • **Continuous evaluation:** Regularly assess the impact of mindfulness on DEI efforts and adjust strategies accordingly • **Setting realistic timelines:** Recognize the need for sustained commitment to see the impact of mindfulness on DEI efforts

Implementation

Implementing mindfulness like any other initiative takes some resources (often around time and incentives) and motivational momentum to encourage buy-in. Speaking of hierarchies, having team and systemic leadership fully on board with the initiative is essential. Successfully implementing mindfulness programming requires a holistic approach:

Education and Training: Offer workshops, courses, or resources to educate healthcare professionals about mindfulness, its benefits, and how to integrate it into their daily routines.

Supportive Environment: Create an environment that encourages mindfulness by designating quiet spaces, providing resources, and emphasizing its importance in staff well-being. Healthcare staff can integrate brief mindfulness exercises into their daily routines to manage stress and enhance focus. Before starting their shifts or during breaks, engaging in a short meditation session can help clear their minds, promote emotional resilience, and increase their ability to cope with the demands of the profession. Group training in gentle movement practices like stretching, QI Gong, or Tai Chi can help us alleviate physical tension caused by long hours of standing or repetitive tasks.

Mindful Leadership: Leaders can model mindfulness behavior, creating a culture that prioritizes self-care, emotional intelligence, and effective communication. Many groups, cognizant of the hierarchies (medical leadership, allied clinical staff, office/administrative staff) find benefit in cultivating "champions" for each of those subsets of the team to mentor and model practice and its benefits.

Integration into Patient Care: Incorporate mindfulness practices into patient interactions, whether through active listening, guided breathing, or incorporating mindfulness techniques into treatment plans.

Regular Practice: Encourage regular mindfulness practice among healthcare providers, enabling them to experience the benefits firsthand. Medical offices and clinics can offer group mindfulness sessions for both healthcare staff and patients. These sessions can be led by trained professionals or through the use of digital resources like meditation apps or online classes. Group mindfulness practices create a sense of community and support among participants, fostering a positive and cohesive environment within the healthcare setting. Moreover, organizing mindfulness workshops and seminars can provide education and resources to staff and patients, promoting a better understanding of the benefits of these practices and how they can be incorporated into daily life.

Sustaining the Initiative: Continuously assess the impact of mindfulness programming through feedback mechanisms, adjusting strategies as needed. Scheduled convening of stakeholders (leaders, champions, and others involved to give "street-level" feedback of the initiative) is important for continued reinforcement and adjustments in expectations and resources.

The buy-in may sound easy, but as we've discussed prior, our temperamental tendencies toward quick outcomes can make medical leadership prone to skepticism about implementation. Setting appropriate timelines for sticking with an implementation plan—think a year at a minimum. Teams may consider one of a variety of validated rating scales about mindfulness to measure progress and identify gaps in implementation.

In Conclusion: Real Team Mindfulness

A truly mindful healthcare system plan integrates self-awareness, empathy, effective communication, and ongoing support to create a holistic approach that benefits both patients and healthcare providers. By prioritizing these elements, healthcare organizations can cultivate a culture of mindfulness that enhances the overall quality of care and sustains the well-being of those within the healthcare system. A successful mindful healthcare system plan recognizes the importance of ongoing education and support. This involves providing resources and training opportunities for healthcare providers to continually develop their mindfulness skills and stay updated with best practices. Moreover, offering mental health and wellness programs can help healthcare professionals cope with the unique stressors of their profession, promoting long-term well-being. Again, this training can be good for the work, and the worker and workplace.

Yet mindfulness employed simply as a therapeutic technique or productivity booster offered optionally or at leisure may fall short of creating true, system-wide impact. By reframing wellness initiatives, such as meditation, creative expression, and social interaction as positive, stress-reducing challenges to incorporate into one's daily schedule, as opposed to self-indulgent activities that detract from patient care, healthcare workers will feel rewarded when accomplishing these challenges, as well as a sense of self-efficacy toward the growth of the overall system. This leadership quality can transform a workplace culture dominated by worry, fear, judgment, critical thinking, and ego-driven personality and behavior into one of growth. Such an environment allows escape from the chronic stress cycle, allowing individuals to grow cognitively and acquire new skills, be more resilient, and be less likely to give up on tasks or blame others for their failures.

By weaving mindfulness into the fabric of health teams, clinics, and systems, a transformative shift toward a more empathetic, patient-centered, and resilient healthcare environment can occur. The result is a win–win situation where healthcare professionals operate mindfully with each other and in our daily clinical work, and patients experience improved well-being and better outcomes. Mindfulness fosters compassion for others and the world beyond, which can be applied directly to work, including social responsibility and environmental sustainability.

We should start early. Incorporating mindfulness training into healthcare training programs from the start offers the invaluable benefit of equipping future healthcare professionals with essential tools for stress management, resilience, and patient-centered care, fostering their overall well-being and enhancing the quality of healthcare delivery. It deserves a place in undergraduate curricula, as well as medical training programs, reinforcing self-awareness from the outset of our training alongside understanding basic science, taking a pulse, listening for a bruit, and tolerating cafeteria coffee at 3 am. After a tough surgery. Realizing the call pager was left in the O.R…

Mindfulness in training programs is our next topic.

Key Points
- Like individual professionals, healthcare teams face both external and internal stressors, and the potential impact of workplace stress on competence, communication, and care.
- Team-based mindfulness practices can be a cost-effective and low-risk intervention that can improve self-awareness, communication, and well-being among healthcare professionals—improving healthcare team dynamics, enhancing collaboration, and preventing burnout among team members, as well as leading to better patient outcomes and a more compassionate workplace.
- Mindfulness can also play a crucial role in addressing issues of diversity, equity, and inclusion (DEI) in healthcare by promoting self-awareness, empathy, and reducing reactivity. Integrating mindfulness into healthcare systems and training programs can lead to a more empathetic, patient-centered, and resilient healthcare environment, benefiting both healthcare professionals and patients.

References

1. Burns LZR, Pauly MV. Big med's spread. MIlbank Q. 2023;101(2):283–324.
2. Royan R, Pendergrast TR, Woitowich NC, et al. Physician and biomedical scientist harassment on social media during the COVID-19 pandemic. JAMA Netw Open. 2023;6(6):e2318315. https://doi.org/10.1001/jamanetworkopen.2023.18315.
3. Spritz N. Oversight of physicians' conduct by state licensing agencies. Lessons from New York's Libby Zion case. Ann Intern Med. 1991;115(3):219–22. https://doi.org/10.7326/0003-4819-115-3-219.
4. Yepes-Rios M, Lad S, Dore S, Thapliyal M, Baffoe-Bonnie H, Isaacson JH. Diversity, equity, and inclusion: one model to move from commitment to action in medical education. SN Soc Sci. 2023;3(3):61. https://doi.org/10.1007/s43545-023-00650-6. Epub 2023 Mar 11. PMID: 36937456; PMCID: PMC10005912
5. Thompson P. How mindfulness helped a workplace diversity exercise. Harvard Business Review; 2017.
6. Goldman Schuyler K, Watson LW, King E. How generative mindfulness can contribute to inclusive workplaces. Humanist Manag J. 2021;6:451–78. https://doi.org/10.1007/s41463-021-00120-2.

Chapter 8
Mindfulness in Healthcare Training

In this section's survey of the variety of roles that mindfulness can play on the professional side of the healthcare ecosystem, we've covered the gamut of its applications and benefits. The profound impact of mindfulness practices on a range of aspects of our profession can make it an essential component of comprehensive patient care and our own self-care.

That survey has included:

- The benefits of **individual mindfulness programming** for us—improving our clinical competencies, interpersonal interactions with both patients and colleagues, and our overall personal well-being in the midst of an ever more stressful workplace.
- The benefits of **mindfulness training for medical teams** in professional settings (offices, clinics, and systems)—improving our communication, collaboration, and care provision; and with benefits in an increasingly collaborative and diverse workforce.

As with our review of the spectrum of tactics and benefits for our patients in entraining mindfulness, the intention is to fully illuminate this foundational human capacity. The adoption of mindfulness into mainstream healthcare has nevertheless been an incremental, even stubborn process.

There are several reasons in play for this slow integration. Our evidence-based rigor can make more empirically vetted approaches like meditation harder to gain acceptance. That some professionals still have limited awareness of mindfulness, or persist in a narrower view of it as a mystical or esoteric practice, has made gaining greater validity and acceptance for mindfulness in mainstream medicine a challenge to date.

Tactically, integrating yet another process and conceptual frame into an already oversubscribed work schedule and set of expectations is a tall order for us, perhaps even taller for mid- or later-career health professionals with long-cultivated and reinforced practice patterns. The intention and hope of the authors is that nevertheless we've generated substantial proof of the benefits of mindfulness to open the minds of our colleagues across the professional spectrum.

The path to adoption for one of the authors (Dr. Sazima, a later-career professional) has taken a more incremental path, initially tiptoeing into mindfulness practices as a low-risk, high-reward adjunctive treatment for patients with psychiatric and chronic medical suffering. That one elder cancine can learn some new tricks is some proof of concept for those of us already somewhat settled into our professional ways.

For the other author (Dr. Chand, an early career professional), mindfulness has been an integrated, parallel aspect of medical training and practice, first discovered during the medical school years and refined throughout the remainder of residency, fellowship, and early independent practice career.

Drs. Chand's and Sazima's shared view is that to truly and fully realize the benefits of mindfulness, the integration of practice should begin right from the inception of medical training and ideally even before, during one's youth. By instilling these techniques early, we believe students will be able to grasp the inherent empathy, compassion, and competent patient-centered care ideals reflected in the four pillars of medical ethics [1]. Those pillars—doing good, doing no harm, patient autonomy, and fairness—can be interpreted as mere esoteric concepts. Yet it takes years of experience in medical training and practice to understand a sense of purpose and ownership in patients directing decisions about their lives, what it actually feels like to "do good" and even "not do bad," and how to feel with our hearts that all living things around us share the same source and are equal beings, worthy of value and respect.

In this context, the importance of mindfulness training at the very beginning of medical education cannot be overstated, as it holds the potential to revolutionize the healthcare landscape for the better. It is not hyperbole to suggest that we can ultimately transform the way healthcare is delivered and experienced, in a moment in which our work is under unprecedented threat.

Mindfulness from the Start: Good for the Training, Good for the Trainee

Interpreting the abundant evidence of benefit, implementing mindfulness in healthcare education may be obvious. But in the setting of a legacy of scientific rigor and historical adherence to educational tradition, change comes slowly and only with time and experience. In our view, implementing mindfulness in this healthcare ecosystem involves two core intentions, perhaps simplistically seen as "heart and head":

- **Heart:** encouraging and building trust in a more direct attention to conscious experience, in the service of our "heartful" intention to be of compassionate service to the suffering and wellbeing of individuals seeking our help.

- **Head:** entraining a set of tactics in mastering, teaching and embodying the trainable, human capacity for mindfulness, in the service of enabling our trainees to better manage their own self-care.

Apart from the future benefits for our trainees in cultivating and complementing competence and fulfillment in the career yet to unfold, mindfulness can be an essential tool for medical and nursing students and allied professional trainees in the **navigation of the demanding training gauntlet** itself. In the three prime areas of benefit of mindfulness practices, we've covered in other areas of the system—attention for **cognitive mastery**, improvement in **interpersonal interactions** with patients and professional peers, and the improved cultivation of sustained **empathy and compassion** in the work—it's hard to argue with early implementation of mindfulness practices.

- The early adoption of mindfulness practices can have a positive, immediate impact on the **intense learning process** in medical training curricula. Mindfulness can be a valuable tool for medical, nursing, and other healthcare trainees in mastering the initial flood of complex medical concepts. By cultivating mindful awareness, students can enhance their ability to focus, concentrate, and engage more attentively with the challenge of our curricula. All of us who have undergone this training can relate to the psychological stress involved in the amount and pace of study and examinations, not to mention the inevitable competitive aspects of training with our temperamental peers—with our high drives and expectations for performance and achievement. Mindfulness encourages a nonjudgmental approach to thoughts and experiences, allowing students to explore difficult or unfamiliar medical concepts with greater patience and an open mindset, especially alongside others. Ultimately, by incorporating mindfulness into study routines, medical students can foster a conducive learning environment that promotes clarity, comprehension, and a deeper understanding of medical knowledge, as well as a natural sense of and striving for collegiality.
- We can view mindfulness in training via a variety of metaphors—as a lifesaver in the midst of a deluge of learning to be done; as a toolbox in managing the shifting emotional states we encounter in the training path; and even as a shield and arrows we use to battle the many challenges in our rigorous and demanding educational sequences. We can also understand ourselves more deeply through the striking and weakening of strong points in our egos, refining our contemplative thought process (as opposed to aimless mind wandering). In these different ways, mindfulness can help us more intimately understand those medical ideals as they relate to ourselves and our interactions with our patients. While these benefits surely impact positively in the midst of training, they also prepare trainees for future adaptability in their careers to come—improving coping, if not pre-empting burnout, in our profession in its current crisis of stress.
- Adoption of mindfulness practices from the outset of training can also play a pivotal role in **enhancing interpersonal skills**. It is perhaps a poorly kept secret that many trainees in medicine, dedicating a decade of our early adulthoods to

deep immersion in intense study and work, may pay a price in underdeveloped adult social skills. The intense focus on academics, long hours, and the emotional toll of dealing with life-and-death situations can limit opportunities for socializing and personal growth during a critical period of life. It can be challenging to form meaningful relationships, balance work–life demands, and engage in non-professional social activities and relationships both during training and then afterward as practicing healthcare professionals. Addressing this issue requires a broad approach, including mindfulness-based strategies to foster healthy personal development alongside our professional training.
- Mindfulness tactics can also help trainees develop greater insight into perspectives outside our own—a foundational skill in "adulting." An individual's ability to become more attuned to our emotions through self-awareness cultivates further development of self-compassion and the ability to soothe and diffuse interpersonal conflicts, which is a sine qua non to molding a positive culture in the workplace. Mindfulness promotes active listening, which is crucial for effective communication in healthcare settings. Such practices can divert young clinicians away from ego-centrism and narcissism and instead toward healthy self-esteem based on our authentic connection to ourselves and with others.
- While mindfulness training shows merit in all three of the realms indicated, perhaps its most potent effect is on the **development of empathy and compassion.** These attributes are integral to the practice of medicine and cannot be overstated—nor adequately learned via textbook curricula. Empathy is closely linked to compassion; careful apprehension of the suffering of others allows for our compassionate response, both in practice and in life. Mindfulness directly fosters our trainees' abilities to better understand our own emotional responses and judgments and those of our patients and colleagues. Trainees can realize early on through direct experience that patients respond better to healthcare providers who are more attuned and attentive to our patients' needs—improving patient outcomes and helping patients feel more cared for and supported. As has been noted earlier, mindfulness can seem alien to other more concrete aspects of medical training. As such, the "better care" intention is the most accessible argument to make.
- The "better communication and interaction" intention is not far behind. The "cultivate compassion" intention may feel the most novel as a trainable "curricular aspect"; even as it is conceptually a sibling to intentions to cultivate a professional outlook based on empathy, ethics, and compassion. These ideals are currently managed preemptively in the residency selection process, then usually discussed and modeled by faculty. Then we hope for the best. Implementing mindfulness training as a formalized, experiential approach to this cornerstone of a healing profession is novel but adjacent.

In these basic ways—**competence, communication, and compassion**—mindfulness practices can supercharge professional development. They deserve a foundational place in all healthcare training programs.

And some students are arriving already tuned in.

Mindfulness at the Outset of the Training Pathway

A fully inclusive implementation plan for mindfulness training should include some appreciation of individuals' premedical training familiarity with and/or actual grounding in mindfulness. There is aggregate data showing tremendous growth in mindfulness practices in the overall US population over the last 10 years [2, 3] (from around 8% in 2012 to an estimated 15% currently)—and in children and adolescents (from under 2% in 2012 to over 7% in a 2017 study, that study published before the explosion in popularity of app-based meditation training since 2018).

Perhaps the broadest medium for exposure to mindfulness tactics is located on the ever-present smartphones of most children, adolescents, and young adults. There is a proliferation of meditation apps, and within those apps a wide variety of sequenced programs and "a la carte" guided practices. An explosion of use of these apps over the last 5 years has followed; 2020 data indicated over 50 million downloads of the top 10 apps. By 2023, the top two apps (Headspace and Calm) combined for 170 million downloads and over 8 million paid subscriptions.

Mindfulness has also become more mainstream in K-12 elementary and secondary education as an effective social/emotional learning tactic. In addition, mindfulness practices as adjuncts to development of spiritual growth have gained popularity in youth groups of most religious traditions as well as in secular humanistic communities.

Undergraduate education is the next echelon of exposure and training, with virtually every college and university offering training curricula as well as access via student health services for the purposes of stress management and self-care. We can even posit that some measure of proficiency in mindfulness or awareness could be included in medical school applications in the future.

Nevertheless, exposure to any and all of this training is not homogeneous, with familiar and unfortunate gaps in access due to financial and racial inequities in educational curricula and access to hardware and Internet access among the prime causes. So while many new entrants in healthcare training may have some familiarity with mindfulness or even any active practice coming in, others may have little or no exposure. This needs to be taken into account in curriculum design.

As noted, our training journey involves Socratic learning that entrants starting medical school are quite familiar with from the structure, if not the pace, of undergraduate studies. While most undergraduate programs celebrate a metaphoric "culture of inquiry" that cultivates intellectual curiosity and discipline as lifelong beneficial processes, training in healthcare is unique in the attention and honor paid to our professional guild and its compassionate ethos. That "heart" aspect of the medical training path is perhaps less familiar to recent graduates from collegiate pre-med tracks. Our culture of empathic awareness and care is a different kind of cultivation, and not routinely formalized in medical schools but rather cultivated by mentoring and modeling from educators and practitioners. Mindfulness education can help from the outset in a more overt attending to the essential mission and outlook that we aspire to as healers and attendants to human suffering.

Mindfulness Programming in Training: General Points

Mindfulness training can and should be integrated throughout the medical curriculum, starting from the beginning didactic work in preclinical years and continuing into and through internship and residency programs. This integration can and has been implemented in a variety of ways.

Dedicated formal lectures and workshops specifically on mindfulness are common, beginning with an introductory lecture set or course on mindfulness, offered early in the preclinical curriculum. The concepts, principles, and scientific evidence supporting mindfulness can be offered in a structured and periodic didactic format. Workshops focusing on stress reduction and self-care using mindfulness techniques can be offered alongside didactics and also be utilized to teach and enforce the basic principles of practice. This can be supplemented by written, audio, and video content.

Sequential/longitudinal training programs can be offered that incorporate mindfulness practices throughout the remainder of the preclinical curriculum. These sessions can be utilized to provide guided mindfulness practices to introduce students to different techniques such as focused attention, breath awareness, and body/self-scanning. As has been reiterated throughout this book, didactics on mindfulness should emphasize its utility for patient care and also for optimizing our own competence, empathic skills, and compassion as professionals.

At best, these discrete educational pathways can be presented in a package, to assure adequate/optimal coverage of this (for now) novel aspect of medical education. An all-in-one approach is more complete but can also risk a failure of adoption. Especially if there is an initial lack of buy-in from faculty, mindfulness training may be marginalized, as can be seen in some other "corners" of our healthcare curricula (nutritional health, mental health, palliative care, and preventive medicine as some common examples).

An alternative or complementary approach to this "bundling" of mindfulness training into a subset of the curriculum is to **integrate the tenets and tactics of mindfulness into existing curricula, lectures, and workshops**. Mindfulness can be incorporated within clinical skills and communication courses, teaching students scenario-specific methods to cultivate mindful presence during patient and collegial interactions, and enhancing empathy and active listening skills. Such courses can utilize role-playing exercises and simulated patient encounters to apply mindfulness in challenging clinical scenarios. Programs may facilitate regular mindfulness sessions where students reflect on patient encounters and explore their emotional responses, which may further provide prompts for individual contemplation or journal entries that foster self-awareness, empathy, and professional growth.

This approach has some advantages. Recruiting and involving current educators in considering and including mindfulness tactics in their own subject matter presentations can reinforce a fuller "buy-in" from our educators in their own education about and adoption of mindfulness. It also has the advantage of modeling and reinforcing its integration in that particular subject matter, both in the particular circumstances of stress management for patients with the conditions being elaborated on, as well as in our own mindful approach to diagnosis and treatment of those conditions.

A drawback to the "fold it into your talks" approach is, ironically, adding an additional mandate to educators, both on the uninterested and perhaps less fair on the interested and well-meaning, who may face an extra burden with no meditative experience. Those of us in educational roles are ourselves wrestling with overall time constraints and dilemmas on how to squeeze an expanding knowledge base into our lectures and workshops. "Add a slide or a case study on how mindfulness relates to your topic and tack on a short, easy group exercise" nevertheless may not seem like too big an intrusion and can hopefully generate its own wave of learning and interest for faculty without a pre-existing familiarity with mindfulness. At best, it can foster new learning for educators and further model mindfulness and compassion in our interactions with students—helping to reinforce a culture of empathy and kindness.

Training programs can also incentivize informal gateways to independent mindfulness practice as our trainees progress through higher levels of clinical education. Students can be encouraged to incorporate mindfulness practices in study breaks, as well as other study skills workshops and wellness programs. Training programs can offer free or discounted subscriptions to mindfulness apps. Providing a designated and outfitted quiet space at training program sites for meditation and reflection is also beneficial.

Mindful Engagement in Educational Settings

Mindful engagement in medical training involves the intentional cultivation of mindfulness practices such as meditation in the midst of classes and workshops, to enhance the effectiveness and wellbeing of our trainees. By incorporating mindfulness into medical education, students learn to manage stress, improve focus, and foster empathy—crucial skills in our demanding and emotionally charged field. Mindfulness also encourages reflection on clinical experiences, helping learners develop a deeper understanding of patients' needs and their own reactions to challenging situations. Ultimately, the integration of mindful engagement in medical training not only benefits the mental and emotional health of future healthcare professionals but also improves patient care by fostering more compassionate, attentive, and resilient practitioners.

The basic science classes all offer the opportunity, either individually or as a class, to begin with a body scan or focused breathing. Every such exercise is a fresh opportunity for students to check-in on themselves and their current state, possibly bringing to light specific emotional responses to a particular curriculum or settling the breath and mind following a stressful event and prior to engaging in new subject matter.

Following such a grounding or zeroing exercise, the array of basic science classes offers a vast, "point-of-care" library of opportunities for mindful application.

Early in anatomy class, we can encourage students to approach cadaver dissections with mindful observation and breathing, gamifying mindful attention alongside deepening the understanding of anatomical structures. The nature of the anatomy lab makes it a perfect, controlled playground to point the mind and breath away rumination and distraction. Dissections, with all their sensory details, textures, shapes, and appreciation toward the gift of human donation, are a setting to practice both focused attention, as well as open monitoring meditation. We can encourage students to practice present-moment awareness during dissection by focusing on their breath and tactile sensations, examining their patience, and whatever may arise during careful removal of fat and exposure of fascia. Incorporating guided reflections after each dissection session to explore the emotional aspects of working with cadavers can also help cultivate empathy.

Returning to our theme of understanding mindfulness as a physiological science in Chap. 2, students can be encouraged to approach their physiology reading and labs with open curiosity and nonjudgmental observation. Time can be allocated for reflective exercises that incorporate meditation where students explore the concepts learned in class and contemplate the interconnection between such physiological processes, their impact on the body, and the broader implications for human health and disease. How such exercises may be crafted and appear, either for individuals or groups, is remarkably variable and left to the eye of the beholder.

Higher-level basic science classes that beg an understanding of granular, at times esoteric, level of information such as biochemistry, genetics, microbiology/immunology, pharmacology, and pathology provide potential scenarios to tie focused attention or open monitoring to the myriad of pathways and reactions that need to be memorized. These years should serve as a preparatory "how to learn" to be a doctor phase as much as they are "what to learn," priming students with meditative techniques to remove moment-to-moment roadblocks as they search their fund of knowledge, approach diagnostic reasoning, and explore potential treatment options.

There are undoubtedly other examples of the application of this "force multiplier" in the basic science years. Safeguarded in the comfort of apartments and libraries during and away from 3 am alarms and uncertain span of hours of the hospital wards, the first 2 years are an ideal setting to embed mindfulness into the rigor of students' daily learning routine, setting the stage for its application in more clinically focused years.

Mindfulness in Clinical Years (Residency, Internships)

Mindfulness training holds particular significance in medical residencies and clinical healthcare internships, now more than ever. This seems especially true in higher-stress specialties, such as emergency medicine. Yet a large nationwide study done in

2012 [4] showed burnout rates almost as high in primary care (internal and family medicine) professionals; and a more recent study [5] concluded that "significantly higher burnout rates were found among female physicians compared with their male counterparts, primary care physicians compared with physicians in other specialties, and physicians with ten years of experience or less compared with those with more experience."

Yet implementing and sustaining mindfulness training in medical residencies and internships presents some obvious challenges. The demanding nature of medical training often leaves little time for additional activities, making it difficult to find dedicated slots for mindfulness sessions. As noted above, there can be resistance from both faculty and residents who may view mindfulness as unrelated to clinical skills, leading to skepticism or lack of enthusiasm. The subjective nature of mindfulness can make it challenging to assess its impact quantitatively, which can hinder its integration into a traditionally evidence-based medical education system. Finally, sustaining mindfulness programs can be challenging due to budget and time constraints. Despite these obstacles, the potential benefits of mindfulness training in terms of stress reduction and improved well-being make it a valuable addition to this "finishing step" in medical education. Finding ways to overcome these challenges is crucial to its successful implementation.

The ideal mindfulness learner in residency is one who has already engaged the concepts and practices optimally during their undergraduate or medical school education. The dilemmas here for residency training programs include the reality of a range of familiarity or lack thereof in incoming residents and healthcare interns in nursing and allied health training. It's likely, then, that while mindfulness-based resilience programs should be available for residents, residencies need to meet our trainees at varying levels of familiarity.

As it does in the clinical sphere, residency transitions to an opportunity to learn mindfulness "on the job." In addition to the workshops, structured meditation groups, and peer support/mindful mentorship from faculty that can be carried over from the basic science years, the clerkship years offer essentially an infinite number of applications of more "practical" mindfulness, especially as it relates to novel forms of stress and anxiety. Continuing from the first 2 years is the key theme of "flexible experiential learning" under a model that readily provides access to guidance from experienced peers. As learners graduate in clinical competency, so too should they be seen as higher-level support structures, able to coach underclassmen through their own mindfulness journey.

Organizing mindfulness segments or workshops as an aspect of resident retreats where students and residents can immerse themselves in intensive mindfulness practice would help solidify weeks and months of individual practice and help learners transcend to different levels of capacity and awareness. To facilitate these immersive learning experiences, invitations can be extended to experienced mindfulness teachers or collaboration with mindfulness centers can be made.

Mindfulness in Clinical Training Settings

Integrating mindfulness training into medical residency clinical rotations offers a multitude of benefits to both residents and the healthcare system at large. Mindfulness practices can provide residents with early career training in valuable tools for stress management, emotional regulation, and resilience building. Our residents can cultivate the capacity to stay present, maintain focus during critical patient care moments, and develop a greater sense of empathy and compassion for their patients, holding true to Osler's definition of "equanimity" for physicians and maintaining calm during the residency storm. It can help faculty model effective teamwork and communication among healthcare professionals. Here are some examples:

- **Rounding:** Beginning Morning Rounds and welcome the quiet of the clinical day with a brief mindful exercise, such as a mindfulness meditation, deep breathing, or a moment of silent reflection helps set a mindful intention, enhances self-awareness, and promotes a focused and compassionate mindset for patient interactions. We can encourage team members to take advantage of mindful pauses, focusing on the breath or body sensations, to center themselves before entering a new patient's room or starting a new clinical task. The end of morning rounds can then be a reminder to partake in a brief "bookend" mindful moment and reinforce a mindful approach to transitions throughout the day, such as between patient encounters or clinical tasks.
- **Patient Care Events:** We can incorporate mindfulness into the physical examination process by guiding residents to be fully present and attentive during patient encounters. We can model the importance of maintaining a compassionate connection while performing physical examinations. The physical examination serves as the perfect opportunity to begin the entrainment of appropriate breath monitoring on our patients. Explaining the secular patterns practice to the patient ("I would like to now describe how I will carry out a mindful physical examination and how you can partake in a calming breathing exercise at the same time") would be a good place to start; inspection (visualization, scanning not only with the eyes but allowing anything to come to you welcomed with curiosity and without judgment), palpation (employing mindful touch alongside focused attention and open monitoring), auscultation (taking the unique opportunity to have a microscopic level examination of the patient's breath or circulatory system, truly being able to identify how it flows, or lack thereof, providing the opportunity for joint breathing entrainment in every single encounter), percussion (a return to mindful touch and an opportunity to close the physical encounter with gratitude). The mindful encounter can seamlessly enter into a review of examination and results, perhaps utilizing a brief 30-s to 2-min breathwork exercise to make the transition. The review of the results and the ensuing discussion themselves are a stage for concerted awareness between doctor and patient. The reveal can often be difficult for patients to handle, making such strategies that can remove barriers toward providing important information or asking important questions.

- **Charting:** Integrating mindfulness into the documentation process helps by encouraging students and residents to approach patient charting with focused attention and nonjudgmental awareness, allowing them to build a positive relationship with the lifelong companion and treat it less as a foe or obstacle in the routine of the day. We can target those moments of extreme annoyance or fatigue when sitting in front of a computer and the only thought on one's mind is to be in the company of their family. We can train our bodies and minds to adapt to the importance of mindful documentation in maintaining accuracy, clarity, and reflection on patient encounters. Such an approach will help clinicians embrace the positive features of such IT systems as they relate to patient outcomes.
- **Communicating:** Integrating mindfulness practices into communication skills training helps by emphasizing active listening, nonjudgmental observation of verbal and nonverbal cues, and mindful responses. We can teach residents (and their medical students on rotation) to engage in mindful pauses during conversations to refine our thoughts and perform mindful contemplation regarding the issue at hand, regulate emotions, and respond empathetically.
- **Shift changes and other workday transitions:** Following morning rounds, shift changes, and call handoffs, mindfulness practices can be encouraged during team huddles to foster a collaborative and supportive environment, as well as remove obstacles that may serve to hand off inaccurate and harmful data. We can routinize beginning huddles with a brief mindful exercise to center team members, promote active listening, and enhance collective decision-making.
- **Closing the day:** The end of a medical resident's workday is a unique, familiar experience all its own in our training gauntlet. The accumulated stress from juggling patient care, complex medical decisions, and long hours often weighs heavily on our trainees. "Landing the plane" from that intensity is its own challenge, often accompanied by the anticipation of preparing for the next day's challenges, and creating a palpable sense of emotional and mental fatigue. These sequences of intensity/brief respite/repeat are really unlike most other civilian professions—and particularly underscoring a need for effective strategies such as mindfulness in our training programs. All faculty, students, and residents may model and encourage engagement in regular personal mindfulness practices to support their well-being, resilience, and ability to provide compassionate care.

Voluntary or Compulsory?

Where might mindfulness training fit in regard to the inevitable "need to know" vs. "nice to know" spectrum? The availability of formal mindfulness training in medical schools may vary from one institution to another. According to a 2017 [6] study, most medical schools (79% as of 2014) have integrated some mindfulness training into their curriculum, while 27% identified formal academic centers devoted to mindfulness training and/or research. That data does not differentiate between voluntary offerings and compulsory attendance. Other schools offer optional courses or workshops on mindfulness and meditation for medical students. Many if not most offer minimal or no training.

The ubiquity of mindfulness practices in virtually every major spiritual/wisdom tradition can militate against individuals protesting the training as a threat or provocation to one's own spiritual value set. Understanding the core benefits—competence, communication, and compassion—and hewing to a secular approach to mindfulness training curricula could and should be reasonable proof of the basic benefit and serve as a counterpoint to any concerns about challenges to individual belief systems.

In that spirit, as mindfulness and its training have broadened mainstream cultural and clinical acceptance in the public domain, having cursory knowledge about it is best considered a compulsory addition to introductory healthcare training programs, including medical schools, nursing schools, and allied health professional training programs. Put another way, the absence of some basic expertise in the concepts and practices of mindfulness is increasingly considered a gap in our professional skillset.

While there is no compelling any of us or our colleagues to personally sustain a meditation practice (nor any other beneficial activity, such as regular exercise or optimal nutrition), we should expect a minimum competency in this validated capacity for self-care. A consensus consideration would be to **include basic mindfulness teaching and some experiential training as a compulsory aspect in medical, nursing, clinical psychology/LCSW/MFT, and allied health professional programs.**

With that initial exposure to the basics of an arguably mainstreamed area of both academic inquiry and widespread awareness, we can respect the developing wisdom and autonomy of advanced trainees (MD residents and fellows, BSN candidates, and interns in psychotherapy and allied health programs) with some choice. "Finishing"/clinical programming can offer mindfulness training in an elective way but offer and model it as a curious and contemplative continuation of that initial compulsory learning and experiential immersion.

Sharpening the Message

Robust resources are available for mindfulness training, as have been identified in detail. Hopefully, there is also a closing gap around the evidence-based proof of mindfulness and its beneficial effects for professionals. Yet perhaps a more useful way to frame the initial approach to trainees is to define mindfulness training in terms of practical solutions to everyday practice challenges, reducing misinterpretation and vagueness.

Our framing of the practical benefits in enhanced attentional control, improved interactions with patients and colleagues, and in cultivating our empathic/compassionate qualities—in shorthand, our three C's of "competence, connection, compassion"—hopefully can provide leaders and exemplars in training programs with a pithy value proposition for championing mindfulness training. These are more concrete targets, eschewing the flow-like training directions of "gaining it, losing it, regaining it," or of tipping toward the more esoteric or New-Age pitches made for training in the broader consumer market.

Mindfulness Training in Nursing and Allied Professional Programs

The implementation of mindfulness training in nursing and allied health professional training programs has gained significant traction in recent years, undoubtedly due to the growing recognition of its potential benefits in the areas that have been reinforced above. Adding additional tools for patient care and education as well as a developing capacity for our own healthy self-care are obviously applicable to all, regardless of our particular role in the healthcare ecosystem.

While our survey of mindfulness in medicine has focused more fully on physicians (such is the perspective of the authors), the implementation of mindfulness training in programs for colleagues in nursing, nurse practitioner, physician assistant, and all other patient-facing allied programs (phlebotomy, technicians in radiology, hemodialysis and others) is equally important, if not more so. As healthcare delivery becomes more stratified and physicians are moving by time pressures and market forces into more assessment/treatment/consulting roles, non-MD professionals are more and more likely to have the most time and direct interaction with patients. From the initial "rooming" and vitals-taking to at-discharge support and education in hospital environments, these settings and situations may often be the optimal time for mindfulness to play a beneficial role, with non-MD professionals in the lead position to provide explanation and some initial training. These colleagues can also use that expertise in peer-to-peer training and support, as was alluded to in the last chapter on mindfulness in team settings. While they are crucial in care provision, by incorporating mindfulness into training, nurses and allied health professionals are also better equipped to cope with these same high-stress environments.

The implementation of mindfulness training in allied health professional and nursing training programs does not need to vary much from that of the other programs discussed. A typical structured approach may include direct lectures and workshops and folding mindfulness content into existing content. Some institutions may offer formal Mindfulness-Based Stress Reduction (MBSR) programs—as described in Chap. 3, typically spanning 8 weeks with guided mindfulness practices, group discussions, and assignments, adapted for healthcare students and with the goal of developing champions of mindfulness within the department. With the importance of clinical application training, applying mindfulness tactics such as the "core 4" (mindful breathing, body/self-scanning, visualization/rehearsal, and gratitude/compassion) to real-world clinical scenarios is a sensible emphasis in initial clinical setting training.

Faculty Training

The effectiveness of mindfulness programs is also reliant on the acceptance and value of clinical teaching faculty. The legacy model of medical education underpins the importance of training faculty members and facilitating a top-down influence of mindfulness from educators to learners. Mindfulness training for faculty members in medical education is essential for fostering a supportive and mindful learning environment. Nevertheless, patience among faculty champions toward incremental acceptance is a preferable approach.

For trainees, faculty members already and inevitably serve as models of self-care, work–life balance, and self-compassion—or not. Faculty members may be trained in mindfulness techniques not only for their own benefit but also to be able to understand how such measures support residents' well-being and resilience. Mindful practices should encourage us to demonstrate active listening skills and encourage open dialogue, nonjudgmental feedback, and compassionate communication among each other and with our trainees.

Taken a step further, faculty can become leaders in mindful clinical teaching practices, emphasizing present-moment awareness and nonjudgmental observation during rounds or clinical procedures. Alongside such practices, dedicated time should be devoted to opportunities for faculty and residents to engage in reflective discussions on mindfulness in clinical practice. By modeling mindful behaviors and emphasizing self-care, faculty members can promote the importance of mindfulness in medical education.

Faculty members should also be offered introductory workshops or sessions to familiarize themselves with the concept and benefits of mindfulness. Resources should be provided, such as literature or online courses, to facilitate a deeper understanding of mindfulness practice and at least support, if not lead, mindful initiatives in the classroom and clinical workspaces. When practical, structured mindfulness-based training programs can be organized, such as Mindfulness-Based Stress Reduction (MBSR), tailored for faculty members. These programs can include guided meditation sessions, mindful movement exercises, and discussions on integrating mindfulness into their professional and personal lives, emphasizing the importance of them serving as champions in the workplace and instructors for their students. Just as for students, regular mindfulness practice groups or other resources can be established for faculty members to sustain their mindfulness practice. Furthermore, participation in faculty mindfulness retreats or workshops could deepen our understanding and commitment.

In addition to clinical performance, faculty members in medical education can hold a pivotal role in rigorously evaluating the impact of mindfulness practices within the training environment. Their unique position allows them to implement and observe the effects of mindfulness in diverse settings, from the structured confines of the classroom to the dynamic and often unpredictable world of clinical wards. By integrating mindfulness exercises into classroom lectures, incorporating mindful reflection in homework assignments, and facilitating mindful practices during clinical rounds, faculty can gather a wealth of data on the effects of these practices on student well-being, resilience, and learning outcomes. Moreover, faculty members can leverage their daily interactions with trainees to initiate mindfulness-based research projects, exploring how regular mindfulness practice influences stress management, decision making, and empathetic patient care. Through these initiatives, faculty can contribute significantly to the growing body of evidence supporting mindfulness in medical education. By conducting well-designed studies and publishing their findings, they can substantiate the benefits of mindfulness, thereby encouraging its wider adoption in medical training programs worldwide.

Integration of mindfulness into and alongside the medical education curriculum is heavily reliant on the support and modeling behaviors of the faculty. Incorporation of mindful techniques, such as brief guided meditations or mindful breaks, during lectures, small group discussions, or clinical rotations, would require full collaboration. Such collaboration would also promote a psychologically safe environment where faculty members and students feel comfortable expressing their thoughts, concerns, and emotions, as well as encourage open discussions about stress, burnout, and the importance of self-care to reduce stigma and promote support-seeking behaviors. Faculty members need to be provided with resources on mindfulness, such as books, apps, or online platforms, to support their ongoing mindfulness practice. Designating dedicated mindfulness spaces within the institution, where faculty members and students can engage in mindfulness practices or take short breaks, would be ideal.

Medical School Exemplar: Monash University School of Medicine, Melbourne

An example of a comprehensive approach to mindfulness training in a medical school training can be found in the mindfulness curriculum of the School of Medicine at Monash University in Melbourne, Australia. Its founder and coordinator, Craig Hassed, trained as a general practitioner and is currently a professor at their Centre for Consciousness and Contemplative Studies. He has fostered the development of Monash's mindfulness programming since the late 1980s.

His 2021 paper, "The Art of Introducing Mindfulness into Medical and Allied Health Curricula [7]," serves as both a road map in terms of content and a pragmatic strategy guide culled from his 20-plus-year work in implementing mindfulness into an existing medical school training program. The paper richly describes the lessons, dilemmas, and some solutions to the process of preparation, integration, delivery, and review of mindfulness curriculum. Under Hassed's direction, Monash first incrementally integrated some mindfulness content and practices into their core medical curriculum starting in the early 1990s. A more thorough and structured curriculum was fully implemented coinciding with a full curriculum update project at

Monash in 2002. From that starting point, the program now educates over 7000 students yearly in medical, nursing, and allied health training.

At the core of the curriculum is a six-week course, taught in the first year of medical school, that combines Socratic teaching and experiential/workshop work, as well as expectations for individual meditative practices. Introductory lectures emphasize the rationale, relevance, and mind-body evidence for mindfulness training and tactics.

The course is notable for its experimental components via individual practice and group discussion.

These include assigned inquiries into students' understanding of perception, nonattachment to phenomena, acceptance of felt experience (as opposed to reflexive judgment), and presence/persistence of mindful awareness. Reflective journaling through the course is mandatory (but not graded).

A variety of direct meditative practices is another central experiential aspect of the course.

- Brief formal practices (dubbed "fullstops") start with 5-min trials twice daily, then advance to 10-min exercises after 2 weeks.
- Brief transitional practices (dubbed "commas"), lasting 15 s to 1 min) are indicated during the learning day, in between scheduled classes and activities.
- Other informal "mindful/mindless" self-checks are reinforced also, driven by inquiry into impacts of various experiences in class as the program proceeds.

The results of this comprehensive training in terms of mindfulness practices "sticking with" future professionals are impressive. In a follow-up survey [8], around 90% of students reported continuing some application of mindfulness in individual practice and as a recommendation in patient care.

Monash's project has also yielded some important lessons that Dr. Hassed elaborates on. These include:

The "pitch" to program faculty/leaders: As also manifest in this book's approach, an assumption that mindfulness and its training may be poorly understood or misunderstood by colleagues is prudent to anticipate. Training terms should be practical and scientific— not New Age or dogmatic/religious. In framing context and rationale, he suggests reinforcing the evidence base for its practical benefits— better care, fewer errors, better communication, and compassion.

Besides the framing of improved clinical competencies, there is value in engaging the self-care, anti-burnout aspect of mindfulness training. Reinforcing self-care as a mandate of good training may run counter for some to the counter-dependent, super-human tropes still prevalent in some of our colleagues, and likely more so among older faculty trained in legacy worldview. The argument can be alternately framed as "we're no good to others if we break down"; and "we model good health for our patients." Ultimately, it's still valid to note that "it can help our trainees, don't you agree?," with no other secondary goal necessary.

Dr. Hassed urges being flexible with the formula to launch an introductory trial/project, albeit with minimums on what can achieve some productive outcomes.

Training the trainers: Programs will optimally need to recruit an initial cohort of faculty to be trained in the curriculum. Participating faculty obviously need to understand and support the core concepts of mindfulness and embody them via practice. Dr. Hassed also infers that while attending to the skeptical among our colleagues is necessary, faculty already practicing mindfulness based in personal spiritual or New Age outlooks may color their teaching from a non-secular stance. Aiming for a shared, consistent approach, faculty are best advised and trained to adhere to mindfulness in medicine in a secular capacity only.

Measuring Effectiveness

Throughout the entire training continuum and its various professional roles, self-assessment tools can be implemented to measure trainees' individual benefit from personal mindfulness practices while in the training sequence. To evaluate the impact both qualitative and quantitative measures may be employed:

- **Validated instruments targeting mindfulness** itself, such as the Mindful Attention Awareness Scale (MAAS) [9] and the Five Facet Mindfulness Questionnaire (FFMQ) [10] can be used, measuring index changes in mindfulness skills and attitudes.
- **Self-report surveys and questionnaires** can assess changes in stress levels, burnout, resilience, empathy, and overall well-being. Standardized instruments such as the Maslach Burnout Inventory and the Jefferson Scale of Empathy can provide valuable insights into the effectiveness of mindfulness interventions.
- **Observational assessments** provide another valuable view of the practical integration of mindfulness into clinical practice. Direct observation of physician–patient interactions, utilizing tools such as the Consultation and Relational Empathy (CARE) measure [11], can assess the impact of mindfulness on communication skills, empathy, and patient satisfaction.
- **Feedback** should be encouraged on the effectiveness and relevance of mindfulness integration in the curriculum. This is best used to refine and adapt our mindfulness training programs based on learners' needs and preferences as stresses and changes. Conducting qualitative interviews and focus groups with trainees and faculty can provide in-depth insights into their experiences with mindfulness training. These interviews can explore the perceived benefits, challenges, and practical applications of mindfulness in medical practice.

The data may also be used for research studies to evaluate the impact of mindfulness integration on trainee well-being, empathy, and patient outcomes.

- **Objective assessments,** including neuroimaging techniques like functional MRI, can examine the neural correlates of mindfulness and its impact on cognitive processes, emotional regulation, and attention. These measures provide

objective evidence of the physiological changes associated with mindfulness practice.
- **Patient feedback and satisfaction surveys** can offer valuable insights into the impact of mindfulness-trained physicians on the patient experience. Assessing patient perceptions of physician empathy, communication, and overall quality of care can provide evidence of the positive influence of mindfulness on the patient–provider relationship.
- **Longitudinal studies** tracking medical students from the beginning of their training through residency and into their professional careers can provide valuable insights into the long-term effects of mindfulness training. By assessing outcomes such as burnout rates, job satisfaction, patient outcomes, and career longevity, these studies can demonstrate the sustained impact of mindfulness on physician well-being and patient care.

In Summary: Mindful Medical Training

Formally implementing mindfulness into the wide spectrum of our various healthcare training programs is a crucial step toward addressing the well-being of professionals and improving care for our patients. By integrating mindfulness throughout the curriculum with evidence-driven rigor, our programs can equip future care professionals with the necessary tools to navigate the challenges of our challenging, rewarding profession. By embracing mindfulness as an essential component of medical education, healthcare leaders can foster a culture of self-care, empathy, and excellence in medical practice.

It also helps develop another, broader human capacity, if one that is not always appreciated. Implementing meditation alongside the rich experiences encountered throughout our medical education pathways—beauty, death, wonder, heartache, joy, and serenity—can also increase motivation and a sense of purpose. It can encourage personal growth and make our relationships more satisfying. It can reduce our own fear of decline and death, and sharpen our passion for a life of meaning and compassionate service. Toward these aspirations, we can begin right from the outset of the journey to mobilize all of our resources in service of this path. With this beginning, mindfulness through meditation and other practices can guide individuals through the rest of their professional and personal lives. Motivated by these transcendent values, as our students become healers, they will have a vision beyond themselves and be better able to integrate all of the sweep of life, accept different perspectives, open themselves to challenges, and truly be aware of the uncertainty inherent in this precious human experience (Table 8.1).

Key Points
- Mindfulness can play a significant role in medical training, benefiting both trainees and the healthcare system. It can improve cognitive mastery, enhance interpersonal skills, and cultivate empathy and compassion among medical students, ultimately leading to better patient care.

In Summary: Mindful Medical Training

Table 8.1 Mindful training, mindful trainee

Key insights	Practical implementation
• Heartful intention: Embraces conscious experience and compassion in healthcare service. Mindfulness nurtures a deeper connection with patients, enhancing trust and empathy • Headful mastery: Mindfulness tactics boost cognitive skills, aiding in mastering complex medical concepts. It allows trainees to absorb knowledge with clarity and focus, vital for effective medical practice • Stress management: Medical training is intense. Mindfulness practices mitigate stress and anxiety, crucial for maintaining mental health and academic performance • Interpersonal skill development: Many trainees sacrifice social skills for academic focus. Mindfulness enhances emotional intelligence, improving communication, conflict resolution, and empathy • Empathy and compassion cultivation: Beyond academic prowess, empathy is the soul of healthcare. Mindfulness deepens understanding of emotional responses, enriching patient care and interactions • Holistic approach to training: Integrating mindfulness into healthcare education is a multi-dimensional strategy. It balances professional and personal development, ensuring well-rounded healthcare professionals	• Curricular integration: Embed mindfulness training in medical curricula. This involves workshops, guided practices, and reflective exercises to ingrain mindfulness habits • Faculty role modeling: Educators embody mindfulness, demonstrating its benefits in practice and teaching. This inspires students to adopt similar practices • Peer support groups: Encourage mindfulness study groups, fostering a supportive learning environment. Shared practices amplify the collective benefit • Assessment and feedback: Regularly assess the impact of mindfulness on students' Well-being and academic performance. Feedback mechanisms help tailor the program to student needs. • Ongoing practice: Encourage students to maintain regular mindfulness practice beyond the classroom. This ensures long-term benefits in their professional and personal lives

- The implementation of mindfulness in medical education should start early, ideally before medical school, and should accommodate variations in trainees' prior exposure to mindfulness practices. Mindfulness programming in medical training should begin early in the curriculum, integrating lectures, workshops, and practical exercises throughout preclinical and clinical years. The integration can either bundle mindfulness training or incorporate it into existing curricula, emphasizing its relevance to patient care, stress reduction, and self-awareness for medical professionals.
- Mindful engagement in medical education enhances students' stress management, focus, empathy, and overall well-being. It can be applied during basic science classes, clinical rotations, and clinical tasks, fostering a compassionate and resilient healthcare workforce.
- The implementation of mindfulness training in healthcare education programs, including medical schools, nursing schools, and allied health professional programs, is increasingly considered a compulsory addition to introductory training due to its potential benefits in enhancing attentional control, improving interactions with patients and colleagues, and cultivating competence, communication, and compassion skills.

- Faculty members in medical education should also receive mindfulness training to foster a supportive and mindful learning environment, promote self-care, and serve as models for trainees.
- Measurement of the effectiveness of mindfulness integration should include self-assessment tools, self-report surveys, observational assessments, feedback from trainees, objective assessments like neuroimaging, patient feedback, and longitudinal studies to track the long-term impact of mindfulness training on healthcare professionals' well-being and patient care.

References

1. Gillon R. Medical ethics: four principles plus attention to scope. BMJ. 1994;309(6948):184–8. https://doi.org/10.1136/bmj.309.6948.184. PMID: 8044100; PMCID: PMC2540719
2. Wang C, Li K, Gaylordd S. Prevalence, patterns, and predictors of meditation use among U.S. children: Results from the National Health Interview Survey. Complement Ther Med. 2019;43:271–6.
3. Kane R. How many people meditate in the world? (2022 Data) | Mindfulness Box. Mindfulness Box, 11 Feb. 2022. mindfulnessbox.com/how-many-people-meditate-in-the-world/
4. Shanafelt MD, et al. Burnout and satisfaction with work-life balance among US physicians relative to the general US population. Arch Intern Med. 2012;172(18):1377–85.
5. Ortega MV, Hidrue MK, Lehrhoff SR, Ellis DB, Sisodia RC, Curry WT, Del Carmen MG, Wasfy JH. Patterns in physician burnout in a stable-linked cohort. JAMA Netw Open. 2023;6(10):e2336745.
6. Barnes MD, et al. An examination of mindfulness-based programs in US medical schools. Mindfulness. 2017;8:489–94.
7. Hassed C. The art of introducing mindfulness into medical and allied health curricula. Mindfulness. 2021;12(8):1909–19.
8. Hassed C, de Lisle S, Sullivan G, Pier C. Enhancing the health of medical students: outcomes of an integrated mindfulness and lifestyle program. Adv Health Sci Educ Theory Pract. 2009;14:387–98.
9. Brown KW, Ryan RM. Mindful attention awareness scale (MAAS) [database record]. APA PsycTests. 2003. https://doi.org/10.1037/t04259-000.
10. Baer RA, Carmody J, Hunsinger M. Weekly change in mindfulness and perceived stress in a mindfulness-based stress reduction program. J Clin Psychol. 2012;68(7):755–65. https://doi.org/10.1002/jclp.21865.
11. Mercer SW, Maxwell M, Heaney D, Watt GC. The consultation and relational empathy (CARE) measure: development and preliminary validation and reliability of an empathy-based consultation process measure. Fam Pract. 2004;21(6):699–705. https://doi.org/10.1093/fampra/cmh621. Epub 2004 Nov 4. PMID: 15528286

Chapter 9
Mindful Technology

"Mindfulness," with its references to ancient wisdoms and a vague interior capacity of individuals, may seem like an unusual term to juxtapose with "technology," having its own associations to futurism and artificiality. "Jumbo shrimp," or perhaps "thank you in advance for this short hold for a pre-authorization representative" comes to mind, oxymoronically. Yet as technology advances in its capabilities to revolutionize healthcare in a myriad of diagnostic and therapeutic ways, it also inevitably intersects with the capacity of mindfulness.

With the COVID-19 pandemic contributing to the acute digitization (the process of converting and storing information into machine-readable data, including data processing, transmission, and combination) [1] of healthcare, and other cultural shifts reflecting the changing nature of the workplace, an expectation of remote working and flexible working hours have become the norm. This shift is finding its way beyond administrative roles and into the provider side of medicine, at least for those specialties that allow for effective clinical remote work.

This digitalization has inevitably led to its own reductionistic model of all things electronic within healthcare's varied and specific niches. Each may promise an acceleration in efficiency and growth. Yet concerns also grow—over information system security behaviors, problematic and addictive technology use, loss of control over technology-mediated decisions, "techno-stress," privacy concerns, and blurred work-life boundaries [2].

Studies are beginning to explore a digital approach to mindfulness training, indicating expanding support and interest. In particular, a 2023 study by Wrede et al. [3] addressed this research gap by exploring how mindfulness and digitalization interact in the digital working context, conducted through qualitative interviews with experts in the field.

The study highlights characteristics of the current digitized workplace to consider:

- **Digital Stress:** The "VUCA" world (volatility, uncertainty, complexity, and ambiguity) of contemporary, tech-driven workplaces leads to a "PAID" reality (pressured, always on, information-overloaded, distracted) for individuals at work. Technology, including hardware and software, acts as both an enabler and a stressor in this context.
- **Implications for Digital Workplace Conditions:** The digital workplace is characterized by a fast-paced environment, increasing task complexity, and blurred boundaries between work and private life. Technology, while offering flexibility and independence, can also amplify stress reactions. Experts point out the stress-inducing aspects of technology, including the "digital hamster wheel" and the challenge of maintaining focus amidst constant digital interruptions. Adjustments in digital work routines are necessary to compensate for digital stress. This involves reducing digital stressors to create room for essential skills like creativity and empathy, thereby fostering innovation.

The study also examines technological solutions to the dilemma, including mindful technology:

- **Mindset and Organizational Culture:** A growth mindset, as opposed to a fixed mindset, is crucial in adapting to digital changes. Mindful attitudes can help organizations navigate these changes more effectively.
- **Mindfulness Practices:** Mindfulness is practiced both formally and informally, ranging from several times a day to cyclically. Mindfulness practice triggers a biopsychosocial relaxation response, reactivating resources and releasing individual human potential. This has positive implications for interpersonal communication, making mindfulness beneficial yet challenging to implement in work settings.
- **Technology as a Catalyst for Mindfulness:** Digital solutions, including on-demand coaches and virtual agents, can free up space for mindfulness practices. Wearables and web-based mindfulness programs with engagement strategies are also explored.
- **Mindful Design:** This theme reflects the need for mindfully designing digital workplace conditions. It includes digital support for meditation and technological innovations such as reminders, blockers, and apps to encourage mindfulness. Technology should be designed to minimize harm to physical and mental health and support formal mindfulness practices at work. The goal is to design technology that is less invasive and more peripheral, to reduce distraction and support mindfulness.
- **Limits of Digital Mindfulness:** The study identifies a "tipping point" where reliance on digital devices for mindfulness can become counterproductive, fostering competitive behavior and possibly leading to excessive reliance on technology.

A recent 2023 systematic review [4] points out that, as it is today, most of where mindfulness and technology practically intersect is in tech's ability to facilitate training for certain patient populations and hypothesizes that smart technology can continue to alleviate many of the challenges currently associated with traditional practice, especially for those with mental health issues.

This discussion is timely in the midst of the concurrent expansion of artificial intelligence (AI), and particularly of the transition from analytical AI, which processes existing data to provide insights, to generative AI, which creates wholly new appearing content or data based on "learned" patterns. The explosive development of generative AI has become an inevitable element of contemporary life going forward, poised to play an ever-increasing role in shaping our future. It is emerging as a transformative tool in mental health programs, offering innovative, accessible, and personalized methods for coaching and therapy. Many other realms of work and society are feeling vulnerable to, yet interested and invested, in the AI movement; ultimately the whole world is tuning in.

In this chapter, we'll expound on the intersection of health/mind and tech in two ways:

- How mindfulness can positively impact our optimal use of the varieties of current and future technologies at our disposal as health professionals—including the risks and rewards of those interactions.
- How technology can be put to use to enhance the entrainment and sustained cultivation of mindfulness, beyond its current applications in apps and other media, by the sound and effective use of AI in applications for both our patients and ourselves.

We can start with that first crossing: our interactions with technology.

Technological Mindfulness

Healthcare professionals have been early adopters of technological innovation throughout history. The record runs back to rudimentary surgical instruments in the Egyptian era, the forerunners of our modern scalpels, forceps, and other tools. The stethoscope, widely identified today as an icon of the profession, was revolutionary when René Laënnec conceived of it in 1816. And some tech has barely changed over the millennia; behold the humble Neti pot, a holdover from early Ayurvedic medicine yet a helpful device still found in chain pharmacies across the globe.

Today's medical technologies are obviously advancing at a velocity that would have been hard to fathom just 40 years ago. Complex imaging tools pinpoint disease with remarkable precision. Genome-driven advances have transformed immunotherapies for cancer and other illnesses. Electronic health records (EHRs), telemedicine platforms, and wearable health devices are just a few more examples of the technologies that have become integral to modern medicine. These technologies ideally enable us to access patient data more efficiently, collaborate with colleagues remotely, and provide more accurate diagnoses and effective treatments.

But medical technology can have marginal, even detrimental effects when engaged mindlessly. We can observe errors in both "commission" and "omission."

On the "commission" side: technology can be a maddening intrusion for many of us, spending our precious clinical minutes staring at screens, re-inputting/cutting/pasting data, and navigating the resultant output from others. The supposed value-add in leveraging our technology can lead into rabbit holes of make-work to appease administrative and medico-legal deities. The time and energy wasted in the haystack-needle searches through mounds of EHR data is an ironic antithesis of the promise of technology to streamline and supercharge our energies and competencies.

On the "omission" side comes what we could be doing in service of our patients instead of data generating and mining. The human touch and empathic interaction that is (or used to seem) crucial to practice gets compromised when we become too absorbed in the digital aspects of our work. Many healthcare settings, recognizing the alienating "look" of the clinician no longer making eye contact with a patient in need of human interaction, but instead furiously typing into laptop templates, have backtracked (pragmatically, but comically) to the use of data-inputting, sidekick "scribes." (Said scribes click-clacking coconuts as they accompany their medical knights into battle could be a Pythonesque touch.)

Sight gags aside, this is the current reality for almost all of us in current practice—a love/hate relationship with our devices, but a dependent one nonetheless. The potential for errors reduced patient interaction, and professional burnout is likely if we cannot find a way to use these awesome but imperfect technologies thoughtfully and effectively. How can we manage it best? As with any individual's relationship with interactive technologies, there are some broader mindfulness strategies and specific tactics that we health care professionals can use to control our tech—rather than it controlling us, via distraction.

First, We Can Sit

The broadest strategy is the most obvious one—cultivating a regular meditation practice. Returning to the core purpose of that practice outlined in Chap. 2, we can engage in the routine of bare observation of our momentary minds, losing that observation in distraction, and regaining that observation. And we can note that this little three-step dance reflects life "off the cushion"—we're tuned in, we get distracted, we regain attention. Even brief but regular practicing of that "attend—lose it—get it back" sequence—yes, over and over—cultivates, over time, a smoother pivot out of distraction, including technological distraction, in our daily work and personal lives. The felt sense of "I'm not really tuned in at this moment" becomes more and more familiar through the simple meditative routine. Or if we are tuned into tech and out of mind, "What am I really giving my precious and vulnerable consciousness and time to?" Through meditation, we incrementally get better at that pivot. That includes pivoting without further inner distraction in the form of judgment about, yes, the distraction itself.

Our professional days are like this, and not just figuratively. That same felt sense we experience in meditation—"aware, then not so much, now I'm back"—inevitably emerges in our daily lives and activities. We fully attend to the medical moment at hand, then lose it into distraction, then regain it. It is experienced for each of us in our very own unique mix of sensation, emotion, thoughts, and our quality of attention. That bespoke concoction can become as familiar in our minds as the feel of motion on our way to work, the awareness of a heart murmur when we listen to a patient's heartbeat, or the empathic pull we feel when a grieving patient tears up in describing a lost loved one to us.

These are all, in short, experiences of a moment in time; our busy professional lives are full of them. The quality of our work really does depend on our sharpened attention in a sea of distractions. More and more, those distractions include technological ones—emails, text notifications of results, patient and peer contacts, and a labyrinthine of EHR platforms. Apart from any other specific tactics we'll review next, a basic cultivation of our own mindfulness capabilities fosters this foundational sense of our own minds as they operate in and out of the fog of distractions.

With a basic mindfulness practice (in whatever form or style it works best) in place, we can also consider some specific tactics to rein in, if not stamp out, distraction-driven mindlessness. These may be familiar from our discussion of the "core four" brief tactics we can educate our patients on: breath awareness for grounding, body/self-scanning, visualization/rehearsal, and gratitude/compassion. We can also pilfer, with gratitude, training tactics implemented at Dr. Craig Hassed's curricula, covered a chapter ago.

"Bookending"

In basic meditation practice, a basic "add-on" to, say, a morning meditation routine, is ending that sitting with some conscious reminder of the aspiration to be as tuned in and aware as possible in the work day/shift/events to follow. It's a simple mental ritual—a word or idea to ping our goal of subsequent mindfulness in the busy day that awaits. It can be "bookended" at the end of the day with another brief sitting to "land the plane," so to speak. That sitting involves generating calm and perhaps some contemplation of the effect of the day, including a sense of the quality of awareness vs. distraction of that work day, now completed. Dr. Hassed's terms of "periods" and "commas" can also apply here, these "bookends" being mental nodal "period" points at which we can attend in quiet, more optimal conditions in opening to experience.

This can be truly helpful in keeping tuned in just before a work day starts, and again at its close. We can even make use of the same technology we're trying to manage, by setting a reminder on smartphones and watches at the appropriate times of day—a ringtone or phrase will do, to remind us we can attend mindfully to what's coming next. It's a brief sensory nudge for a valuable intention.

We can use a scaled-down form of this "bookending" (Dr. Hassed called them "commas") in transitions between activities—in this case, mindful interactions with technology. A couple of breaths, or even a brief scan of body/heart/head/watcher, can precede the flipping open of the laptop, the keying in of an EHR password, or the tapping of the text message icon on our smartphones. When the technological task is completed, "bookend" with another brief, mindful breath or two, or a brief scan. The intention here is mostly about alerting ourselves against falling into some metaphoric place of distraction (rabbit hole, maze, thicket, web... all can apply) in the particular technological interaction. It also serves to combat the fiction of "multitasking," of attempting to attend simultaneously to, say, texts, the screen in front of us, and a conversation. There's lots of evidence that this state of action is built on the mistaken idea that attention is spread, when it's really just frantically, compulsively bouncing among targets. Yet we can easily fool ourselves that we are optimally performing at all of the tasks, or even any of them.

Instead, we can strive to give each task, technological or otherwise, our full attention. That intention is reinforced by a brief "bookend" of a breath or two, centering our attention, leading into a technological task and then out of it. Then on to the next event—and its next opportunity to "bookend" and attend more fully. While conceptually this can seem like extra effort to practice—"How is this helping me become more efficient?"—as with the sequences of basic meditation, the "here's the next task... tune in for a sec first" becomes conditioned in a familiar way and then ultimately second nature, as does the process "bookending" when starting or finishing a task. The proof, even though there is a randomized controlled trial [5] demonstrating that present-focused monitoring skills training drives mindfulness intervention-related improvements in momentary attentional control, which in turn fosters greater trait attentional control, may just be in the pudding. Sorry, in the sitting; when we take off and land the plane in the morning and evening. A practice abound with "bookends" can intuitively be seen as one that ameliorates potential challenges that may arise during dedicated, more formal meditation, and, just as importantly, that helps to aid in the overall acceptance of the practice. The same is true in reverse, as we've touched on [6], that practice of "acceptance" training demonstrates independent improvements in attentional control.

Digital Diets and Detoxes

Getting out of the weeds of momentary experience, we can also impose some broader discipline in our overall time in thrall to technology. As opposed to faddish diet and "detox" regimens, this need not involve, say, cayenne-infused pickle juice or ingesting coffee via unexpected orifices. Instead, some common sense and self-discipline—skills we medical professionals generally have a deep affinity for—can be used effectively. Besides the aforementioned "attend fully to one task" tactic, consider these other obvious, but mindful tactics in engaging with technology:

A **digital "diet"** involves a mindful and intentional approach to our use of technology, aimed at promoting a healthier and more balanced relationship with our digital consumption. Outside the broader daily nudge in meditation to any more tuned into our actions and reactions, we can consider scheduling "mealtimes"—consciously setting aside dedicated times during the day for checking emails, reviewing electronic health records, or responding to messages. Of course, the promise of consolidating our tech "meals" assumes a commitment to, in today's fad parlance, "intermittent fasting," and a reduction in "grazing," often mindlessly, outside of those scheduled events. Obviously, our profession often requires the nimbleness to drop the current for the urgent. But some scheduled moments to directly attend to these aspects of our technological interactions can reduce the building of stress and improve the quality of our responses.

Establishing periods of **"digital detox"** during the workday can help us fully (if briefly) disconnect from technology and reconnect with ourselves and our patients. It provides an opportunity to step away from the relentless notifications, emails, and electronic records, allowing us to clear out mental and emotional clutter and recharge our cognitive resources. This can and already does take the form of identified peers fielding incoming contacts while on hospital rounds, so as to clear the "field" for full attention in patient visits. For ourselves, scheduled breaks in "tech-free" zones, outside the usual four walls—a walk around the grounds of the hospital or clinic, or even a few minutes in a pleasant public area inside a medical complex, such as a lobby, chapel, or designated contemplation room, common in most hospitals. As our days' transition from professional to personal, setting boundaries on technology use in personal life can also contribute to greater mindfulness at work.

While there is no apt comparator to a weight scale or serum "crit level" to monitor our progress in dieting and detoxing from mindless scrolling and searching, some ongoing attention is best paid to how these tactics are being applied and benefited from. Most smartphones, for example, can log hours on screen time used, as one example. Less formally, a quick attending in a brief evening meditative sitting to "How tuned in/out am I today?" is likely to reinforce this aspect of our daily practice. Regularly reflecting on our digital habits and their impact on patient care and well-being can motivate us to make adjustments and strive for a healthier balance between technology benefits and burdens.

Technology can be, as the cliche goes, a blessing and a curse. As we may encourage our patients to take more control of self-care, we can model healthy boundaries in our mindful approach to this aspect of contemporary life. "Bookends" of mindful tuning-in in the transitions of our daily events, portion-sizing of our intake of medical both on and off the clock, and purposeful moments of restraint and engaging the natural and human world "off the screen" are all helpful and easily applicable.

From this discussion of mindful approaches to technology, we'll now invert that phrase and explore technological approaches to mindfulness. How can technology be put to best use in the entrainment and sustained cultivation of mindfulness, beyond its current applications in apps and other media, by the sound and effective use of AI? What would optimal mindfulness technology, particularly tech that health professionals would gravitate to for our patients and ourselves, look like? Understanding the basics of AI is a proper first step.

AI: A Brief Summary of a Complex Topic

As a brief introduction, artificial intelligence (AI) is a broad term that encompasses the development of computer systems that can perform tasks requiring human-like intelligence, including machine learning, natural language processing, and problem-solving. Much of this new technology is driven by "large language model learning," in which computer modeling systems ("models") process massive amounts of data cultivated to date across the web, recognize patterns in language (grammar, context, semantics, etc.) and use those processes to produce coherent and contextually relevant text content (and images and coding, among other content) in return.

Getting just a little deeper into the weeds: with AI, individual data inputs we make into a program or "network" are processed based on the principle of "ground truth"—a data set of existing individual inputs and outputs, based on objective information or data considered to be the correct or most accurate answer to a particular task or problem. With a ground truth established, mathematical functions ("kernels," in AI parlance) process subsequent data inputs, allowing AI networks to generate the most accurate answer to a new question or problem. That data processing also serves to train, validate, and evaluate the AI network, further shaping it going forward.

What separates the newer generative AI movement from the more historical analytical AI is an extra, albeit not completely transparent, layer of "deep machine learning," which is what allows a network to be autonomous in its own learning and adaptation based on prior, existing results of that learning. In other words, an AI network is something that learns in a sustained way and can be modeled and developed for any particular task or purpose.

Amid this complexity, there is debate and concern around the transparency, interpretability, and explainability of AI, particularly those "ground truths." Valid questions about biases, fairness, and ethical concerns that may be embedded in the datasets that generate ground truths are at the center of the debate. As they serve as benchmarks for evaluating the accuracy and performance of AI systems, the selection, curation, and representation of ground truths are critical in reinforcing or mitigating biases and disparities in AI applications. As AI systems increase in complexity, the transparency, interpretability, and explainability of AI—in essence, how these systems can continue to be understood by humans as they further evolve—are important concepts for us to be aware of as AI becomes more widely used in healthcare.

Healthcare leaders are charged with the sensitive task of integrating AI into our profession. AI is ideally positioned to work alongside healthcare professionals for the common good. Yet anxiety, stress, and fear can follow over accuracy, privacy, ethics, and even job security. Reshaping part of our workforce based on AI's capabilities to perform some tasks with similar or better outcomes is one valid dilemma; there are others, beyond the scope of this book. The weighing of the net benefits and risks of using AI to improve healthcare provision for both patients and professionals is just beginning.

One area of early adoption of AI is in medical research, education, and writing. In fact, the production writing of a large part of this book was assisted by the use of generative AI technology. The authors have found benefit in a pragmatic culling of additional information, conceptual frames, and segments of prose using ChatGPT, the most well-known of the current AI platforms. As such, many of the chapters warrant this anodyne statement for AI citation, as many texts currently being produced with the aid of AI technologies for other subjects will certainly require going forward:

> *During the preparation of this work the author(s) used chatGPT, a writing source that uses generative AI technology, in order to generate chapter layout and content specific to the referenced articles. After using this tool/service, the author(s) reviewed and edited the content as needed and take(s) full responsibility for the content of the publication.*

As many other writers and readers have noted, we have found that AI is remarkable in generating information, but not so much just yet in writing style. Our conclusion is to work with AI, yet it like we would any other scientific source, and direct it to help us further our goals in expansion of medical knowledge, like supercharged assistant secretaries [7]. It can also be a powerful tool in providing improved clinical care and, in our case, educating our colleagues about the various uses and benefits of mindfulness in the world of medicine.

Mindful... AI

Diving into the ever-expanding world of digital wellness, a myriad of meditation applications is already available offering a varying range of features designed to guide users toward cultivation of mindfulness. The range of current applications is impressive, yet often adopt a one-size-fits-all approach that reflects a desire for broader consumer adoption. There are some unique challenges in adapting mindfulness tactics specifically to the healthcare sphere. A truly healthcare-specific app remains a niche not yet fulfilled, awaiting a tailored solution that speaks directly to the experiences and needs of both medical professionals and our patients. Furthermore, harnessing the value of appropriately integrated AI can help produce a more organic, developing mindfulness practice, one that grows with the user, both professional and patient. Here we review some functions of a true "mindfulness in medicine""app and how AI can play a role in those functions.

Many AI networks, or "neural networks" as they are termed in the AI sphere, are being adapted for use in smartphone applications, including in apps for mindfulness. The contradictions are obvious: bright, flashy, and eyeball-capturing phone apps would seem to be the epitome of distraction, however, "optimized" with AI technology. Naysayers bound to the Freudian principles of transference and countertransference will amount, raising concern over the physical loss of the psychotherapeutic environment. Yet, leveraging the power of AI to build an optimal mindfulness app for patient use and medical benefit is a legitimately optimistic idea. Can we envision AI as a mindfulness teacher, a psychotherapist, and even a personal assistant for patients and providers alike as they navigate healthcare situations and circumstances … all in one?

Prior to going down any rabbit hole of what an innovative "mindfulness in medicine" application could be, we should first consider and hopefully buy into some "ground truths" of our own. One is that mindfulness "works"—that training this human capacity is truly beneficial for both patients and professionals. With that case made, there is the other buy-in: that AI is here to stay and can be used ethically by healthcare professionals in many productive ways, including in mindfulness training development.

With those two cases made, we can consider what an optimal, AI-assisted mindfulness app could provide, especially beyond what is currently offered in mindfulness apps. There is an ironic similarity in both the machine-learning technology of AI and the interior-learning process of mindfulness training: both learn, albeit in different ways. The shaping of our consciousness—by regular inputs of bare observation in the formal practice of meditation and the informal intention of mindfulness in daily life—is a process of inputs honing and shaping our own "ground truths" to know ourselves better. In AI, inputs are also necessary to continually validate and sharpen the "ground truths" that result in AI networks.

In that spirit, healthcare professionals and our patients (at least those of us with buy-in to the validity of both mindfulness and AI) have an opportunity to provide input both in the big-picture sense and in a literal sense. In a broad way, we have the opportunity to participate in the development of AI-assisted mindfulness training and help pave the way for better diagnosis, treatment, or other big-picture insights, such as chatbot controlled medical trials across thousands or even hundreds of thousands of patients. The more literal sense involves the value-add of AI in any training app: with repeated inputs from the user, the app learns and grows with that user, providing personalized suggestions, tracking progress, and offering real-time feedback in addition to adapting to cognitive and behavioral patterns based on such real-time data.

Mindful AI Technology for Patients

The integration of artificial intelligence (AI) into the implementation of mindfulness practices in tech/app form for patient use can lead to several best-case uses. An AI-enhanced mindfulness app can enhance the effectiveness and accessibility of mindfulness training. Here are some ways in which AI can play a positive role in the individual patient's experience in this context:

- **Personalized Mindfulness Programming and Feedback**: Leveraging AI, the app can personalize meditation sessions based on user preferences and communication of emotional states, offering tailored guidance and content. AI technology can analyze an individual's data inputs, including self-report and rating of stress states and identified emotional responses, even during the use of mindfulness exercises in the app itself (judgments and other thoughts that arise, heart rate, respiration, anxiety, or physical pain experienced).

Real-time feedback and guidance after and even during meditation sessions, through interactive prompts. For example, AI can access a combination of attributes, including facial landmarks, bodily sensor data, contextual attributes, and time duration, to successfully detect human distraction and gently guide practitioners back to present moment awareness.

As interactions and inputs accumulate, the app can analyze user feedback, journal-based and otherwise, and even physiological data (from wearable tech, for example) to provide insights into and suggestions for the user's mindfulness practice. AI can also incorporate natural language processing for guided meditation scripts specific to context. Chatbot-based support to address challenges during the meditative process, should the user desire to troubleshoot them in real time, is another possible innovation.

AI-based pattern recognition can thus allow for a kind of individualized "learning" and development as an individual interacts with the app over time. In this way, a personalized mindfulness program tailored to the specific, changing needs and goals of each person is cultivated, and ensuring that mindfulness practices within the app are relevant and effective for each individual user.

The aforementioned 2023 systematic review by Mitsea et al. extensively highlights the unique opportunities and challenges of digitally assisted mindfulness platforms, a few of which are highlighted below:

- **Telehealth Integration**: AI-powered telehealth platforms can incorporate mindfulness interventions into virtual healthcare visits. As discussed in Chap. 4, brief meditative tactics are useful for patients in preparing for an office visit, managing the stress of bad news during the visit, and concluding the visit. An app-based virtual "mindful assistant" could join the call, knowing names and context, and offer adjunctive support interventions for those key moments and others. This can allow healthcare providers to model such tactics in-visit, even virtually, leading to more openly and successfully prescribed mindfulness practices as part of a holistic approach to medical and mental health.
- **Natural Language Processing (NLP) and Cultural/Language Adaptation for Guided Mindfulness**: AI-driven virtual assistants can engage in conversations with individuals, learning about them and adapting to them over time. Such an app could provide a "pocket psychotherapist," capable of generating empathetic and personalized support and answers for questions, as well as offer guided, personalized, accessible mindfulness sessions. AI can aid in adapting mindfulness practices to various cultural contexts (including alongside other healthcare team members or patients) and languages, making them more inclusive and accessible to diverse populations.
- **Extended Reality (XR), including Virtual Reality (VR), Augmented Reality (AR), Mixed Reality (MR), and the Metaverse**, is transforming mental health

training by offering a range of immersive technologies. VR creates a fully immersive virtual environment, tailored to individual needs and effective in isolating distractions, thus enhancing focus and inducing calmness, especially beneficial for those with social anxiety. It leverages the power of attention for self-regulation and enhances sensory awareness through rich experiences. AR blends real and virtual worlds, aiding those with mental imagery challenges by enhancing sensations, and is accessible through simple smart devices. MR, a hybrid of AR and VR, allows interaction with virtual objects in real settings, bridging virtual and real worlds. The Metaverse offers a persistent, multiuser ecosystem that combines physical and digital realities, enabling embodied interactions in a socially interactive environment. While these technologies are increasingly used in mindfulness training, the effectiveness of XR-based interventions in mental and emotional regulation is still being explored.
- **Data Tracking, Reminding, Summarizing**: AI-based capabilities can track a plethora of data or inputs, vital sign parameters, and total meditation hours for instance, provide a unique, "gamified" experience based on the user, and be able to provide useful summaries of progress and help refine practice areas that need attention. The tech term of art for this is "gamifying": applying game-like elements and mechanics to the practice of mindfulness to make it engaging and interactive, encouraging users to cultivate mindfulness skills while having fun.
- **Predictive Analytics for Medical, Mental and Cognitive Health**: Healthcare firms such as insurers, health systems, and pharmacy benefit management firms are already using AI to analyze historical health data to model and predict which individuals might be at higher risk of increased stress and reduced compliance with individual best practices in managing chronic medical and mental health problems. AI-guided mindfulness interventions can be recommended proactively to prevent or mitigate these issues. The intervention can also be tailored to individuals with cognitive impairments, such as dementia or attention deficits, to improve cognitive function and quality of life.
- **AI-Enhanced Mindfulness Research**: AI can process and analyze remarkably large datasets of mindfulness practice (or other health) outcomes, identifying patterns and insights that can assist the development of more effective interventions, identifying key factors and insights that contribute to effectiveness, and helping refine protocols.

As much as advancement in technology and innovation can help our patients, this same technology can help healthcare professionals in our own work and personal mindfulness training.

Mindful AI Technology for Professionals

For medical professionals, tailored/guided meditation programming can be an accessible and beneficial resource, given the unique contours of our challenges both in training and in practice. Our work often treads upon paths laden with profound interactions, emotional demands, and moments of introspection. One day might bring the joy of a patient's recovery, and the next, the profound sorrow of loss or guilt of errors in practice. Custom-guided meditation exercises based on the "core four" tactics—customizing a visualization or scanning sequence to specific personal contexts are examples—can provide solace in these moments, offering structured narratives specifically designed to address experiences like dealing with the passing of a patient, navigating the complexity of patient relationships, or simply finding calm after a marathon of long work hours.

Our profession thrives on precision and individualized care. In much the same way, leveraging generative AI for meditation practices offers the potential for personalized precision that resonates deeply with each user. Rather than adopting a one-size-fits-all approach, AI-curated meditations delve into the nuanced emotional and mental states of each user. By analyzing an individual's mood and emotional states, any transmitted physiological data, preferences, and current needs, the AI can craft sessions that are not just generic stress-relievers but pinpointed therapeutic sessions addressing specific emotional landscapes. For a surgeon coming off a high-pressure surgery, an intern navigating the challenges of a new environment, or a seasoned physician grappling with burnout, AI can discern the subtle cues and generate a meditation that feels tailor-made. With every session experienced, rated, or provided feedback on, AI learning garners more understanding about the user. This continual interaction allows the refinement of recommendations and personalized strategies over time. It is comparable to having a meditation instructor who gets to know us better with each interaction, understanding our individual emotional and biological rhythms, and adjusting guidance accordingly. Moreover, this feedback mechanism ensures that the AI remains adaptable, continually updating its strategies to cater to changing user needs and preferences.

Designed for the field of medicine, such an application could especially appeal to future health professionals who often strive to demonstrate these capacities in training applications and interviews.

Here are some particular potential programs and benefits:

- **Daily Medical Mindfulness:** Recognizing the constraints of time and the emotional pendulums that medical professionals often swing on, a "Daily Medical Mindfulness" feature can be a set of scheduled prompts and inputs—brief, powerful touchpoints to anchor one's day. Just a few minutes, strategically placed at the beginning and/or end of day, can act as effective "bookends" as noted above, ensuring that each day starts with intention and winds down with reflection.

- Scheduled "**Mindful Break**" exercises can help ground us in the flow of busy work days. Harnessing the power of generative AI, these mindful breaks are not just generic pauses, but finely tuned to the individual needs and preferences of the user. Recognizing the nuances of every medical professional's specific routine, AI technology can craft personalized mini-meditations, guiding the user to breathe, reflect, and momentarily detach from the immediacy of our duties. They are particularly useful for those of us preparing for surgeries, critical procedures, or challenging patient interactions. These practices can help anchor ourselves, focusing minds and steadying hands, centering the collective consciousness of the medical team on the patient and the task at hand. Such practices are not merely about calming nerves but about harnessing our full cognitive, interactive, and empathic potential at critical junctures. A feature of these "mindful breaks" lies in their adaptability—as short as a minute or extended to ten, fitting snugly into whatever gap is available in a hectic schedule. Additionally, as the AI learns more about the user's preferences, patterns, and feedback, the app can refine its recommendations based on those inputs—generating an improving purposeful, personalized interlude, reminding healthcare professionals of the importance of self-care, even in the briefest of moments. A "Daily Medical Mindfulness" aspect is not just about offering sporadic relief but about integrating mindfulness into the very fabric of a medical professional's routine. By doing so, it ensures that amidst the whirlwind of duties and challenges, we can easily access a moment of pause, a touch of tranquility, and a reaffirmation of purpose. Another potential component would leverage the use of wearables like smartwatches.

- An **"Emergency Calm"** feature could provide swift intervention prompts in moments of high stress, potentially linked to the stressful context (exam failure, interpersonal conflict, patient death/suicide, and medicolegal stress). Recognizing the individual's own particular ID of stress triggers and responses, this feature could rapidly assess the user's current emotional state and deliver a tailored, instant meditation or grounding exercise. These interventions, which would last just a few minutes, are crafted to bring the user back to a state of balance, grounding them in the present moment and allowing for clearer, more focused decision making.
- **Mindful Focus:** A suite of AI-driven auditory aids can be offered, crafted via use and inputs to help medical professionals reduce distraction and heighten concentration. At the heart of this component lies the understanding that our brain responds uniquely to different auditory stimuli. What might be a soothing background sound for one might prove distracting for another. This is where the strength of AI-driven customization comes to the fore. Instead of providing a one-size-fits-all solution, the application learns from the user's preferences and patterns. Over time, the app can tailor a soundscape (and added landscape with augmented/virtual reality headsets) that aligns seamlessly with the individual's concentration rhythm, amplifying focus and minimizing the lure of distractions. It can also gauge the optimal volume, pace, and sequence, ensuring the auditory experience is as fluid as it is effective. For many of us, tasks demanding immediate and sharpened attention aren't limited to a particular setting or time—emerging in the middle of a night shift or during a short break between surgeries.

"Mindful Focus" programs provide a tool at their fingertips wherever they are. In a profession where precision is paramount, these enhancers serve as invaluable allies, ensuring clarity in thought and precision in execution.

- **Mindful Movement:** In the relentless rhythm of medical practice, physical well-being can sometimes be overshadowed by the mental and emotional demands of the job. Hours on end can be spent in the same posture—be it bent over an operating table, sitting through long lectures, or standing during ward rounds. Over time, this physical stagnation can take a toll, leading to stiffness, discomfort, or even chronic pain. A Mindful Movement component can meld physical rejuvenation with mindful awareness. Concise, guided exercises within this feature can be tailored specifically for the challenges healthcare professionals face, aimed for effective use in fleeting breaks between patient consultations or surgeries. These mindful exercises can be designed not just to alleviate physical tension, but also to anchor the mind, making the practitioner more present in their body. Examples include a quick session guiding a surgeon through a series of wrist and shoulder stretches, releasing the tension built up from hours of meticulous work; seated spinal twists and neck stretches for radiologists stiff from poring over images; grounding foot exercises, for nurses and technicians needing to feel more rooted after a long shift on our feet. The dual benefit is physiological, for overall bodily comfort; and psychological, serving as a grounding reminder for practitioners to inhabit our bodies fully, even in the midst of external chaos. While the world of medicine is undeniably cerebral, it's crucial to remember the intimate connection between mind and body. The Mindful Movement component emphasizes this union, providing medical professionals with tools that cater to our unique physical demands while simultaneously nurturing a deeper sense of embodied mindfulness.

- **Mindful Community:** Our field, despite being intrinsically interconnected by shared experiences and goals, can often feel isolating. With the challenges that come from long hours, emotionally charged situations, and the weight of responsibility, the need for a supportive, interactive community becomes paramount. A Mindful Community feature should be an aspect of a comprehensive Medical Mindfulness application—a virtual gathering space specifically designed for medical professionals to come together, share their journeys, seek advice, and find solace in shared experiences. The use of AI-guided moderation plays a pivotal role here. While human touch and empathy are irreplaceable, AI ensures that the environment remains conducive to open conversations without the risk of negativity or trolling. It can monitor discussions, flags any potential concerns, and can even suggest resources or interventions if a member seems particularly distressed. This creates a safe haven where professionals can express themselves without apprehension, knowing that the space is guarded against any undue negativity. The Mindful Community component would be more than just a discussion board; it's a lifeline for the end of shift or on-call MD. Providing an avenue for medical professionals to connect, converse, and care for one another reinforces the idea that while the path of medicine might be challenging, no one has to walk it alone. In this digitized era, it serves as a reminder that sometimes, the most potent medicine is the knowledge that someone else understands. The community can represent the user, as well as the institution and represent individual achievements and milestones alike, further serving as a framework for other users and healthcare systems to build from.

Another potential application of AI technology could link aggregate data from users for broader research purposes to target broader stress management interventions for particular specialties, schedules, and sequences in training programming. As mentioned above, Virtual Reality (VR) is yet another emerging technology that could lend itself to a "Mindfulness in Medicine" suite of applications for more immersive stress reduction. Through AI-personalized sessions, medical professionals can access a meditation experience that feels genuinely ours, offering a sanctuary of tranquility and introspection amidst the bustling corridors of hospitals and the relentless demands of our profession.

Caveats

In all of these examples, we can consider a plausible and valuable application of AI technology within the realm of mindfulness and mental well-being. This intersection of technology and well-being promises a future where technology doesn't just facilitate wellness but actively contributes to it. Yet, as with any innovation in our field, some important practical and ethical considerations need to be attended to. Readers are encouraged to visit Mitsea et al's 2023 systematic review of digitally assisted mindfulness (see references) for an extensive outline of challenges associated with digitally assisted mindfulness.

- **Commercialization of Mindfulness:** This development could dilute the power and the genuine benefit of mindfulness practices for user wellbeing—a truly ironic twist. Apps should prioritize benefit over "upselling" poorly devised or trendy features and other profit-driven acts that could undermine trust in the practice and its association with ineffective, artificial, "inauthentic" technological interface.
- **Vulnerable Patient Populations**: The use of AI chatbots in therapeutic settings can be challenging for patients with severe mental health issues, cognitive impairments, or those who have experienced trauma. These individuals may require a level of empathy and understanding that AI currently cannot provide. The risk is that AI chatbots might misinterpret or inadequately respond to complex emotional states, potentially leading to misunderstanding or even harm. There's also a concern regarding privacy and data security, especially for those who may not fully understand or consent to how their data is being used.
- **Lack of Available Research**: Current studies often lack the rigor needed to draw conclusive results about the efficacy of AI in psychotherapy. More high-quality research is needed, focusing on long-term outcomes, the impact on different types of mental health conditions, and how these interventions compare to

traditional therapy methods, including detailed qualitative studies on the implications and challenges of conversing with a nonhuman entity, the loss of traditional transference and countertransference, as well as which digital surrogates may serve in their place [8]. Research should also consider the ethical implications and potential biases in AI algorithms. This research gap underscores the need for comprehensive studies with robust methodologies, possibly involving randomized controlled trials and long-term follow-up to assess the true impact of AI-driven mindfulness interventions.

- **Misuse of Mindfulness Practices:** The "commodification" inherent in a market-driven application could oversell its benefits and lead to its use as a form of escapism or retreat rather than awareness building. Another form of misapplication takes the form of considering such technology as a valid/adequate substitute for robust mental healthcare—rather than a complement to such treatment.
- **Privacy and Security Issues:** These are likely the most front-of-mind concerns for individuals, in or outside healthcare. Sensitive biometric and mental health data collected through AI-driven mindfulness applications could be vulnerable to data breaches and privacy violations. Unauthorized access to users' mindfulness records or personal information would have obvious and significant negative consequences for individuals and undermine trust in mindfulness platforms and applications.
- **Fraudulent "Use" in Treatment and Training**: An accessible app being "prescribed" as an aspect of treatment in medical or mental health settings, or as an expectation for individuals in health care training programs can obviously be misused. There may be a concern that individuals are logging sessions without actually performing practice. Digital display of hours of practice serving as a faulty surrogate marker to focus and compassion. "Going through the motions" sham practice and even outright cheating are valid concerns, but ones that are well-known to traditional mindfulness practice. They don't outweigh its potential benefits, as well as the invaluable, kind resource it presents to those who are interested and committed. Technological adherence "checkpoints" are available in smartphone technology to ensure practice is honestly adhered to.
- **Disadvantaged Patient Populations:** The accessibility of smart technology poses a significant challenge for disadvantaged patient populations. These groups often lack access to the necessary technology and Internet connectivity required for AI-based interventions. This digital divide means that the benefits of such technologies are not equitably distributed, potentially exacerbating existing health disparities. Moreover, disadvantaged groups are frequently underrepresented in research, leading to a lack of data on how these technologies impact diverse populations. Future research and policy efforts need to focus on increasing accessibility and ensuring that these innovative interventions are inclusive and tailored to meet the needs of all segments of the population, regardless of their socio-economic status.

It is essential for us to prioritize ethical AI development in this space, ensure robust data protection measures, and maintain a balance between technological innovation and the core principles of mindfulness, such as self-awareness, empathy, and genuine well-being. Integrating AI into mindfulness practices should be guided by our commitment to well-being, ethical considerations, and a holistic understanding of health—foundational tenets we cherish in the profession as a whole.

In Summary: Mindfulness and Technology

In that intersection of mindfulness and technology lies a promising path in broadly opening out access to many more patients, leveraging technology to spread beneficial mindfulness training far and wide, toward the betterment of both our patients and ourselves. Allowing us to more easily educate our patients in these practices through the latest tech, we can truly collaborate in the shared goal of better health.

By embracing technology-enhanced mindfulness practices ourselves, we healthcare providers can enhance our own professional competence, communication, and care—and our own personal well-being. As these two realms cohere, we have the opportunity to create a healthcare ecosystem where technology supports and amplifies the compassionate and mindful care that patients deserve while safeguarding the mental and emotional resilience of those of us who provide it. It's a synergistic approach that recognizes the importance of the human touch in medicine and leverages technology's potential to augment, rather than replace, the vital connection between healthcare professionals and our patients, ultimately leading to better outcomes and a healthier future for all of us.

Key Points
- The intersection of mindfulness and technology is becoming increasingly relevant, particularly in the context of the digitalized healthcare landscape, where technology can both enhance efficiency and create stressors.
- Mindful strategies for managing technology personally and professionally, "bookending" to start and end tasks with intention, implementing digital diets and detoxes, and exploring technological solutions like AI for sustained mindfulness cultivation.
- Artificial intelligence (AI) encompasses various computer systems capable of human-like intelligence, utilizing machine learning, natural language processing, and problem-solving. Generative AI, empowered by deep machine learning, allows AI networks to learn autonomously and adapt based on prior results. However, concerns about transparency, interpretability, and ethical biases in datasets persist, especially in healthcare applications. Integration of AI in healthcare raises questions about accuracy, privacy, ethics, and job security, with a need to weigh the benefits and risks for both patients and professionals.
- An exploration of an optimal implantation of AI in mindfulness technology for both patients and health professionals includes daily practices implemented through AI-driven prompts and inputs, personalized meditation exercises

generated by ongoing journaling inputs, and accessible/personalized "mindful Break" exercises to provide brief pauses for reflection and grounding.
- Ethical AI development, data protection measures, and a balance between technology and mindfulness principles are crucial for successful integration. Potential caveats include the commercialization of mindfulness, potential misuse of mindfulness practices, privacy and security concerns, and the digital divide in disadvantaged patient populations.

References

1. Ritter T, Pedersen CL. Digitization capability and the digitalization of business models in business-to-business firms: past, present, and future. Ind Mark Manag. 2020;86(0019–8501):180–90.
2. Turel O, et al. Panel report: the dark side of the digitization of the individual. Internet Res. 2019;29(2):274–88. https://doi.org/10.1108/intr-04-2019-541.
3. Wrede SJ, Esch T, Michaelsen MM. Mindfulness in the digital workplace: an explorative study of the compatibility of mindfulness and technology. Research Square; 2023. https://doi.org/10.21203/rs.3.rs-2459776/v1.
4. Mitsea E, Drigas A, Skianis C. Digitally assisted mindfulness in training self-regulation skills for sustainable mental health: a systematic review. Behav Sci. 2023;13(12):1008. https://doi.org/10.1108/intr-04-2019-54110.3390/bs13121008.
5. Chin B, et al. Mindfulness interventions improve momentary and trait measures of attentional control: evidence from a randomized controlled trial. J Exp Psychol Gen. 2020;150(4):686–99. https://doi.org/10.1037/xge0000969.
6. Rahl HA, et al. Brief mindfulness meditation training reduces mind wandering: the critical role of acceptance. Emotion. 2017;17(2):224–30., www.ncbi.nlm.nih.gov/pmc/articles/PMC5329004/. https://doi.org/10.1037/emo0000250.
7. Walsh D. A blueprint for using AI in psychotherapy. Stanford HAI, 21 June 2023. hai.stanford.edu/news/blueprint-using-ai-psychotherapy.
8. Holohan M, Fiske A. "Like I'm talking to a real person": exploring the meaning of transference for the use and design of AI-based applications in psychotherapy. Front Psychol. 2021;12:27. https://doi.org/10.3389/fpsyg.2021.720476.

Chapter 10
Conclusion: Mindfulness and the Future of Medicine

As we conclude this broad review of mindfulness in medicine, we hope the result is an illumination of this capacity that we all have, can cultivate, and ultimately use for the benefit of our patients and ourselves. Our approach to this subject has been informed by our shared appreciation for the practice and is anchored in the need to make an evidence-based argument to our colleagues for the great value of mindfulness in healthcare.

To recap, our case for mindfulness proceeded through these steps:

- We covered the **concepts and definitions of mindfulness as a trainable capacity of the mind**, different types of mindful practices, and the various benefits of mindfulness encompassing somatic, emotional, mental, social/interactive, and spiritual aspects.
- We delved into the **neural mechanisms behind mindfulness**, the role of emotions in the brain, and the impacts of mindfulness on brain plasticity, neuroendocrine function, and immune function. We presented **research on its benefits** for physical health conditions and mental health, providing current evidence supporting mindfulness-based interventions across various populations in healthcare. For our colleagues looking to start mindfulness initiatives in institution, knowing this language is important. We encourage those who are interested to continue paying attention to the most recent mindfulness literature.
- We reviewed the many guided and manualized meditation approaches, provided an introductory **guide to basic breath meditation**, and offered some guidance on our approach to **patient education in mindfulness practices** as well as a summary of various mindfulness-based and related therapies.
- We looked at the many ways **healthcare professionals can incorporate mindfulness into clinical settings and situation**s, tailoring mindfulness techniques to benefit a range of patient populations in both medical and mental health contexts.

- We pivoted from the application of mindfulness tactics for patient care to its benefits for us as healthcare professionals—framing its utility in enhancing the (hopefully memorable) triad of competence, communication, and compassionate care. We covered **our own potential use of mindfulness** in a range of settings, from individual offices to clinics, hospitals, and healthcare systems.
- We made a case for the **inclusion of mindfulness training from the outset of medical education**, integrating mindfulness concepts and techniques into the training of medical students, residents, nursing students, and allied healthcare trainees from the beginning to enhance their education and skills.
- We explored the intersection of **mindfulness and technology**, leveraging the cutting-edge power of artificial intelligence (AI) to address current gaps and limitations in mindfulness training, and enhance customization and accessibility. We emphasized the importance of integrating mindfulness philosophy into mindful AI development and addressing ethical concerns related to privacy, bias, overreliance, and misuse.

Mindfulness is a basic aspect of human experience that has nevertheless been subject to some misunderstandings over time. The diverse cultural and historical roots of mindfulness and meditation as well as its adoption in different contexts have led to various interpretations of mindfulness, some of them limited or flawed.

Our profession rightly draws some bright lines between the perceived secular versus sacred aspects of compassionate care—between "church and state," metaphorically. This distinction is perhaps obvious but is an essential split from the ancient legacy of spiritual and folk healing that predates modern medicine, yet still has its adherents.

Medical knowledge and technological advances are growing exponentially. The foundational, timeless aspect of the compassionate, human relationship between caregiver and the suffering has a different path in terms of its development—less driven by new data, more by openness to new and deeper ways of internal development of our humanity. Excitement about the latest medication or procedure understandably garners less awareness than the patient, incremental development of, well, our awareness.

From the current values and challenges we encounter in today's healthcare ecosystem, what can we expect down the road? And how can mindfulness practices play a valuable role in that future?

We can start from the very first idea in this book: Medicine is at an inflection point, with a paradox of truly remarkable advances in care yet also a true crisis in effectiveness, fair access, and professional burnout. Our field can expect further advances in patient care that revolutionize the way we understand and treat diseases. From groundbreaking therapies to cutting-edge technologies, the potential for improving and saving lives has never been greater.

Yet this continuing era of unprecedented progress is juxtaposed with a harsh reality—a genuine crisis in the effectiveness of healthcare systems, equitable access to these life-saving innovations, and the alarming rise of professional burnout among our community of healthcare providers. The very same medical breakthroughs that hold immense promise also raise difficult questions now and going forward about their affordability, availability, and equitable distribution. And we on the front lines of healthcare, dedicated professionals who tirelessly care for our patients, are facing a relentless and often overwhelming burden—driven by long hours, high-stress environments, and emotional exhaustion. This crisis in professional well-being threatens not only the health and happiness of our community but also the quality of care we provide.

Easy and holistic solutions to this paradox are beyond the scope of this book. We must all hope they are not beyond the scope of our profession and our leaders. Identifying the current problem points is clearer than forming solutions and strategies to implement them in a political and economic era so prone to contention over compromise and hyperbole over common sense.

At first glance, considering the beneficial role of self-awareness practices and concepts, mindfulness included, might appear counterintuitive, unconventional, a leap—especially within the context of a healthcare system wrestling with the massive issues noted. Yet the prospect of transformation in healthcare ultimately resides in the minds and hearts of individuals, of each of us. It is a simple but profound recognition that any change begins with our personal capabilities of awareness and intention. Each of us within the healthcare ecosystem possesses the potential to contribute positively. As has been reiterated through this book, mindfulness encourages us to become more attuned to our own thoughts, emotions, and actions. So it is obvious that mindfulness can help each of us to play a pivotal role in any process of meaningful change.

Mindfulness operates on an individual level, regardless of that individual's position to participate in improving medical care. Yet individual intentions based on compassionate self-awareness can generate waves. When individuals within the healthcare system embrace mindfulness, we can create a ripple effect that can extend throughout the entire ecosystem. A mindful approach to our work can inspire colleagues and peers to do the same. We can foster a culture of empathy, collaboration, and continuous improvement. This cultural shift can lead to the implementation of innovative solutions, improved communication, and a greater emphasis on preventive care and well-being.

With that intention in mind, we can look here at some overall trends to consider in medicine's future, and the future of mindfulness practices. Rigor and common sense demand we have a clear eye about both the optimistic and the troubling trends.

Future Trends in Medicine: Advances and Concerns

According to the analyses of innumerable policy experts, the future of medical care is poised to undergo significant transformations driven by three primary movers: advances in technology, especially using Artificial Intelligence (AI); evolving healthcare delivery models that decentralize care from traditional settings; and a growing emphasis on personalized and preventive medicine. We can touch briefly on each of these and their linkages:

- **Technology advances**, already having transformed much of medical care in the last 50 years, are reshaping the profession at an unprecedented pace. The growing application of technology to make treatment both more personalized and precise includes advancements in genomics, AI-enhanced predictive models for treatment planning, advanced drug therapies, and "smart" wearable and implanted tech devices for both monitoring and care delivery. Perhaps the biggest shift of late, and that will inevitably grow and morph our work, is not medical but in communications: the advent of telemedicine.
- The COVID-19 pandemic accelerated by necessity a huge leap in **decentralizing the provision of healthcare services**, one that will only grow over time. Virtual consultations, remote monitoring of chronic conditions, and digital health platforms offering personalized health information and guidance are obvious examples. That decentralization via technology can at best foster an increasing emphasis on collaboration to reinforce good health.
- That collaboration is essential in our profession's shift toward a **preventive and lifestyle-oriented approach to care.** The emphasis on health promotion, nutrition, exercise, and mental well-being to reduce the burden of chronic diseases and improve overall population health. Especially important is an increased attention paid to nurturing healthy practices early in life, reducing the adverse stresses and traumas of family dysfunction that can deeply impact children and are predictive for a host of subsequent medical and psychological problems later in life.

These areas of change are themselves superimposed on a complex interplay of societal demographic changes and market forces that we cannot expect to ebb. These include:

- **Demographic changes in age and income inequality** are foremost in the dilemmas we must find solutions for going forward. Many countries are facing an aging population and with that, demands for specialized and complex care for chronic and age-related conditions.
- This dynamic can strain healthcare resources already competed for by another challenged demographic: **underserved and poor populations.** This demographic is not monolithic globally but often includes younger individuals for which barriers to healthcare, especially including preventive care and adequate mental healthcare, not only generate current suffering but also increased longer-term need for healthcare resources and, ultimately, poorer health outcomes.
- **Fragmented systems of care** cause overall waste inefficiencies that drain health budgets. These inefficiencies in administration—and perhaps most provocatively, at least for healthcare professionals, the well-intended but often complicating morass of EHR and other IT expectations—waste time and resources. The byzantine system for authorizations, referrals to specialty care, accreted by the web of ever-changing relationships among insurers, healthcare groups, pharmacy

benefit management entities, and others makes for anything but a smooth path for patients and caregivers alike.

Even in the midst of the great promise of developments noted above, the countervailing problems risk the biggest concern for our profession and our patients: a loss of trust in the humanity of our profession. The positive legacy of medicine as a profession of competence and compassion is eroding, and can be difficult to earn back.

That same legacy is under threat for our own community of professionals. Later-career professionals are losing trust in a system that drives over-work and under-appreciation, and especially an intrusion into the human connection we expect with our patients. Earlier-career professionals and trainees are understandably questioning the trajectory of these trends and the impact on their career choices. So, we share an erosion of trust in the humanity of our profession.

But the erosion of the humanizing aspects of medicine is not inevitable.

While mindfulness is no panacea for these challenges, it is a human capacity that should be a part of any solution. These practices can play a pivotal role in humanizing medicine and mitigating the erosion of trust. On the patient-centered side, trust can be rebuilt and sustained if we reinforce mindfulness tactics to foster excellence in the three foundational areas we've emphasized: competence, communication, and compassionate care. On the "provider-"centered side, mindfulness encourages our self-awareness, reducing burnout and enhancing our ability to cope with the pressures of the profession. As a result, the two aspirations can co-create a virtuous circle, working together to restore trust in the medical field, strengthen our relationships, and, ultimately, improve healthcare outcomes.

A Time to Act

This integration is unlikely to happen organically; however, compelling the case can be made for mindfulness' role in healthcare. Here are some concrete actions that we can take to support the integration of mindfulness in our profession:

- **Participate:** This first step is the most obvious one—to take advantage of any mindfulness training programs offered by your workplace, healthcare facility, or local community. Hopefully, this book has generated evidence-based "proof of concept" and useful information on mindfulness' benefits—the first directive in our "see one, do one, teach one" trope. But each of us can experience firsthand the benefits of mindfulness only by direct practice. "Do one," indeed.
- **Educate:** This book has provided a host of possible uses of mindfulness tactics. With some conceptual understanding and direct practice under our collective belts, we can proceed to "teach one," or many. We can support and participate in teaching workshops or seminars for our colleagues and staff to educate them about the benefits of mindfulness and its potential in clinical and personal settings. We can encourage open discussions and knowledge sharing. We can stay

up-to-date with developments in both the mindfulness and AI fields within healthcare.
- **Advocate:** We can spread the news about the breadth and benefit of mindfulness in our work settings and teams, to human resources entities in our larger systems, and through our professional associations to include this training in their guidelines, conferences, and continuing education programs. We can advocate for funding for research, and especially in reducing equity gaps in mindfulness training for underserved communities. Lastly, we can advocate for the responsible and ethical use of mindfulness in healthcare, especially in the burgeoning use of AI and other technologies—emphasizing the importance of maintaining patient privacy and data security. We can encourage an ongoing dialogue on ethical guidelines and best practices.

As with any virtuous project, it takes mindful effort and intention. We all can contribute to the integration of mindfulness in healthcare, ultimately enhancing the well-being of healthcare providers, improving patient care, and advancing our field.

Finally, A Mindful Intention

While our healthcare system may seem vast and unwieldy, meaningful change ultimately begins within the minds and hearts of the individuals who humanize it. The practice of mindfulness empowers individuals to tap into their inner resources. As we individuals collectively adopt mindful attitudes and behaviors, we generate the potential to drive a transformative shift in the entire ecosystem.

Mindfulness in medicine has the potential to revolutionize healthcare. We can bring forth a new era of compassion, efficiency, and well-being for both patients and healthcare professionals.

We can imagine a healthcare ecosystem where physicians, nurses, and our allied clinical colleagues are not only highly skilled but also deeply attuned to the emotional and mental needs of our patients. We can picture a world where innovative technology can assist us in sustaining our competence, communication, and care. We can envision a future where our patients, empowered by mindfulness practices, actively participate in their own healing and health.

We can embrace the promise of reducing our own burnout and sustaining our professional and personal well-being.

This transformation is not merely a distant dream. It's a reality we can actively shape. By advocating for mindfulness programs, supporting research endeavors, and embracing solutions, we pave the way for a more compassionate and effective healthcare system.

In this vision, we find hope and encouragement. Together, we can create a mindful healthcare landscape where humanity thrives.

Key Points
- We conclude by emphasizing the significance of mindfulness in the field of medicine, highlighting its potential benefits for both patients and healthcare professionals, and restating case for incorporating mindfulness into healthcare—with practical applications in clinical settings and integration into medical education.
- The future of medicine is discussed, with a focus on three primary drivers of change: advances in technology (particularly AI), decentralization of healthcare delivery, and the increasing emphasis on personalized and preventive medicine.
- We recognize an erosion of trust in the medical profession and recommend mindfulness practices as a means to humanize medicine and rebuild trust.
- Concrete actions, including participation in mindfulness programs, educating colleagues, and advocating for mindfulness integration, can support its adoption in healthcare and help to build a more compassionate and effective healthcare system.

Appendix A

Scales, Measures, Assessments, and Surveys

The Mindful Attention Awareness Scale (MAAS)

The Mindful Attention Awareness Scale (MAAS) is a well-regarded tool for assessing mindfulness skills and attitudes. Developed by Kirk Warren Brown and Richard M. Ryan, the MAAS is a 15-item questionnaire designed to evaluate open or receptive awareness of and attention to present experiences. It is known for its strong psychometric properties and has been validated in various settings, including with college students, community members, and cancer patients.

The MAAS questionnaire uses a Likert scale, ranging from 1 (Almost Always) to 6 (Rarely), for respondents to indicate the frequency of their experiences. Each statement on the assessment relates to the concept of present-moment awareness. The total score is calculated by finding the mean or average of the 15 items, with a higher score indicating a higher degree of dispositional mindfulness. This means individuals with higher scores are likely more proficient at self-reflection and being consciously receptive to their internal state and external environment.

This scale is not only useful for personal self-awareness but also serves as an effective tool in coaching and therapy settings. It helps individuals understand their baseline level of mindfulness and set future goals for enhancing their mindfulness practices. However, it is important to consider some limitations of the scale, such as the potential for reporting bias due to reliance on self-reporting and the need for more empirical research across diverse demographics.

The MAAS is an effective tool for understanding and developing mindfulness, particularly in clinical and coaching contexts. It allows for a quantitative measure of a subjective experience, providing valuable insights for both the individual and the professional working with them. More information about the MAAS and access to the questionnaire can be found on the Positive Psychology Center's website [1–3].

For more detailed information and to access the scale, you can visit the University of Pennsylvania's Positive Psychology Center website or the National Academy of Sports Medicine's blog [4].

The Five Facet Mindfulness Questionnaire (FFMQ)

The Five Facet Mindfulness Questionnaire (FFMQ) is a widely used assessment tool that measures mindfulness in individuals. It was developed to provide a comprehensive measure of mindfulness, covering five key facets:

Observing: This facet focuses on the awareness of sensations, perceptions, thoughts, and feelings.

Describing: This involves the ability to articulate internal experiences with words.

Acting with Awareness: This facet refers to engaging in activities with full attention and avoiding automatic pilot mode.

Non-judgmental Inner Experience: This involves taking a non-judgmental stance toward one's thoughts and feelings.

Non-reactivity to Inner Experience: This facet is about allowing thoughts and feelings to come and go, without getting caught up in them.

The FFMQ includes both a long-form version with 39 items and a short-form version with 15 items. It uses a Likert scale for responses, and scores can be directly or reverse scored depending on the item. The questionnaire is self-scorable and assesses mindfulness in a broad range of contexts, from general well-being to handling stressful life events. The FFMQ has been validated across diverse populations and has shown strong psychometric properties, including high test-retest reliability and internal consistency. Research has demonstrated its utility in predicting positive thinking, uplifted mood, and subjective feelings of well-being, making it a valuable tool for psychological assessments and mindfulness research.

The FFMQ is available for use in both clinical and non-clinical settings and is suitable for individuals aged 16 years and above. It is effective in determining whether mindfulness practices are enhancing mindfulness over time or if low mindfulness levels could be impacting psychological health.

For further details and access to the questionnaire, you can visit resources like PositivePsychology.com [5] and NovoPsych [6, 7].

Maslach Burnout Inventory (MBI)

The Maslach Burnout Inventory (MBI) [8] is a key tool for measuring burnout, consisting of 16-22 items in five validated forms. It assesses individual experiences across various occupational groups. The MBI-Human Services Survey (MBI-HSS) and the MBI-HSS for Medical Personnel are widely used in healthcare. They evaluate three scales: Emotional Exhaustion, Depersonalization, and Personal Accomplishment. The MBI-General Survey (MBI-GS) is suited for non-healthcare occupations. Items are scored on a 7-point frequency scale, ranging from "never" to "every day," measuring three independent constructs rather than a single burnout scale. Its effectiveness has been proven in numerous studies across different professions.

A study focusing on US attending anesthesiologists post-pandemic era utilized the MBI to assess burnout metrics. The study defined burnout as a high score on emotional exhaustion (greater than or equal to 27) and/or depersonalization (greater than or equal to 10) alongside a low score on the sense of personal accomplishment (less than or equal to 33) [9].

Additionally, the use of MBI in various healthcare settings, including among public healthcare professionals, is the subject of ongoing scoping reviews and research, indicating its widespread applicability and relevance in diverse medical environments [10].

The MBI and MBI Manual are copyrighted publications obtained directly from the publisher at their website: www.mindgarden.com/products/mbi.htm.

The Jefferson Scale of Empathy (JSE)

The Jefferson Scale of Empathy (JSE) is developed to quantify empathy levels in patient care settings. It has been rigorously tested worldwide, demonstrating high reliability and validity. This scale is particularly important in healthcare as it helps assess and enhance empathy among practitioners and students. The JSE has been shown to be sensitive to changes over time, making it useful for evaluating the effectiveness of educational and interventional programs aimed at fostering empathy.

Key findings from research involving the JSE include a study [11] led by Dr. Mohammadreza Hojat at Thomas Jefferson University, which examined empathy in nearly 11,000 US first-year osteopathic medical students. This study found variations in empathy scores based on gender, ethnicity, and chosen medical specialties. The 2018 study examined the measurement properties, underlying components, and latent variable structure of the JSE. The study involved a web-based survey that included the JSE and found significant gender differences in JSE scores, favoring women. It identified three factors of Perspective Taking, Compassionate Care, and Walking in Patient's Shoes. The study also developed a national norm table for assessing students' JSE scores.

The JSE has been used extensively in various studies, affirming its role in improving patient care and supporting the professional development of physicians and nurses. Its broad application and the insights derived from these studies contribute significantly to understanding and enhancing empathy in healthcare.

For more detailed information and further reading on the JSE and its application in healthcare, you can visit the Thomas Jefferson University's website and NCBI.

The Consultation and Relational Empathy (CARE) Measure

The Consultation and Relational Empathy (CARE) measure is a tool created by Dr. Stewart Mercer and colleagues from the Departments of General Practice at Glasgow University and Edinburgh University to assess patients' perceptions of relational empathy during medical consultations. It was designed to be meaningful to patients regardless of their socio-economic background. The development and validation of the CARE measure involved qualitative and quantitative approaches, including correlational analysis against other validated measures and patient interviews. The initial version of the CARE measure showed strong correlation with established empathy measures like the Reynolds empathy measure (RES) and the Barrett-Lennard empathy subscale (BLESS), but subsequent versions were modified to reduce skewness in distribution and improve internal reliability [12].

The scoring system of the CARE measure is based on a scale where each item is rated as "poor"=1, "fair" = 2, "good" = 3, "very good" = 4, and "excellent" = 5. The scores for all ten items are added up, resulting in a maximum possible score of 50 and a minimum of 10. Up to two "Not Applicable" responses or missing values are allowed and are replaced with the average score for the remaining items. Questionnaires with more than two missing values or "Not Applicable" responses are discarded from the analysis [13].

A study published in "Fam Pract" in 2005 by Mercer et al. provided performance data on the CARE measure in a large sample of general practice consultations. This study included 3044 patients attending 26 different practices. It found that the CARE measure was highly relevant to patients' current consultations, with 76% of patients rating it as "very important." The study concluded that the CARE measure is considered by both GPs and patients as directly relevant to everyday consultations in general practice, across both high and low deprivation settings [14].

These studies indicate that the CARE measure is a reliable and relevant tool for measuring patients' perceptions of relational empathy in the consultation, making it a valuable instrument in the evaluation of empathetic communication in healthcare settings.

References

1. Mindful Attention Awareness Scale | Positive Psychology Center. Upenn.edu. 2019. ppc.sas.upenn.edu/resources/questionnaires-researchers/mindful-attention-awareness-scale.
2. Kirk Warren B, Ryan RM. The benefits of being present: mindfulness and its role in psychological well-being. J Pers Soc Psychol. 2003;84(4):822–48.
3. Carlson LE, Brown KW. Validation of the mindful attention awareness scale in a cancer population. J Psychosom Res. 2005;58:29–33.
4. Bender D. Learn how to use the mindful attention awareness scale (MAAS) as a coach. Blog.nasm.org, blog.nasm.org/mindful-attention-awareness-scale.
5. Chowdhury MR. The Five Facet Mindfulness Questionnaire (FFMQ). PositivePsychology.com. 27 Aug 2019. positivepsychology.com/five-facet-mindfulness-questionnaire-ffmq/.

6. Five Facet Mindfulness Questionnaire (FFMQ-15). NovoPsych, 24 Sept. 2021, novopsych. com.au/assessments/formulation/five-facet-mindfulness-questionnaire-ffmq-15/.
7. Baer RA, Carmody J, Hunsinger M. Weekly change in mindfulness and perceived stress in a mindfulness-based stress reduction program. J Clin Psychol. 2012;68(7):755–64. https://doi.org/10.1002/jclp.21865.
8. https://www.researchgate.net/publication/263810021_Maslach_Burnout_Inventory_%2D%2D_Human_Services_Survey_HSS. Accessed 1 Jan 2024.
9. Afonso AM, et al. U.S. attending anesthesiologist burnout in the postpandemic era. Anesthesiology. 2023;140(1):38–51. https://doi.org/10.1097/aln.0000000000004784. Accessed 24 Dec 2023
10. Soares J, et al. Use of the Maslach burnout inventory in public healthcare professionals: A scoping review protocol (preprint). JMIR Res Protoc. 2022;11(11):e42338. https://doi.org/10.2196/42338.
11. Hojat M, et al. The Jefferson scale of empathy: A nationwide study of measurement properties, underlying components, latent variable structure, and national norms in medical students. Adv Health Sci Educ. 2018;23(5):899–920. https://doi.org/10.1007/s10459-018-9839-9.
12. Mercer SW. The consultation and relational empathy (CARE) measure: Development and preliminary validation and reliability of an empathy-based consultation process measure. Fam Pract. 2004;21(6):699–705. https://doi.org/10.1093/fampra/cmh621.
13. Consultation and Relational Empathy (CARE) Measure. The Center for Compassion and Altruism Research and Education. ccare.stanford.edu/rescarch/wiki/compassion-measurements/consultation-and-relational-empathy-care-measure/. Accessed 24 Dec 2023.
14. Mercer SW, et al. Relevance and practical use of the consultation and relational empathy (CARE) Measure in general practice. Fam Pract. 2005;22(3):328–34. https://doi.org/10.1093/fampra/cmh730. Accessed 15 Apr 2019.

Appendix B

Recent Mindfulness Research

For Patients

Effect of Mindfulness-Based Therapy on Spiritual Well-Being in Breast Cancer Patients: A Randomized Controlled Study [1]

This study investigates the impact of mindfulness-based therapy on the spiritual well-being and quality of life of breast cancer patients. Conducted as a randomized, controlled trial with 70 participants from September 2021 to July 2022, the study utilized methods like the Patient Sociodemographic and Medical Data Form and Functional Assessment of Chronic Illness Therapy-Spiritual Well-Being (FACIT-Sp). Results indicated significant improvement in the therapy group's spiritual, emotional, and physical well-being, along with overall quality of life. This underscores the potential benefits of mindfulness-based training in enhancing the well-being of breast cancer patients and suggests its incorporation into nursing practices. The FACIT-Sp measure and licensing opportunities are available at https://www.facit.org/measures/facit-sp.

Mindfulness-Based Stress Reduction (MBSR) Effects on the Worries of Women with Polycystic Ovary Syndrome (PCOS) [2]

This study investigates the impact of mindfulness-based stress reduction (MBSR) on the mental health of women with polycystic ovary syndrome (PCOS). Conducted on 60 women in Iran, the research employed a quasi-experimental design.

Participants in the intervention group underwent eight 90-min MBSR sessions over several weeks. The study's focus was on a range of worries including mental and interpersonal problems, physical complications related to non-pregnancy and pregnancy, sexual complications, and religious issues.

The results demonstrated a significant reduction in the overall worry scores in the intervention group compared to the control group, both immediately after the intervention and 1 month later. This finding was consistent across all six domains of worries assessed by the research. The study concludes that MBSR counseling effectively reduces worries and improves the mental health of women with PCOS. This suggests the potential of MBSR as a therapeutic approach in health centers for patients with PCOS, addressing not just physical symptoms but also the psychological and emotional challenges associated with the condition.

Mindfulness and Relaxation-Based Interventions to Reduce Parental Stress, Anxiety, and/or Depressive Symptoms in the Neonatal Intensive Care Unit: A Systematic Review [3]

The systematic review examines the effectiveness of mindfulness and relaxation-based interventions in reducing stress, anxiety, and depressive symptoms in parents with infants in Neonatal Intensive Care Units (NICU). The review found that these interventions may effectively reduce anxiety symptoms, with moderate to large effect sizes. However, the results regarding their impact on parental stress and depressive symptoms are mixed and less conclusive. The review identifies methodological weaknesses and heterogeneity in interventions and participant adherence as challenges to drawing strong conclusions. Future research is suggested to focus on standardized interventions, diverse parent populations, and rigorous study design to better understand these interventions' effectiveness in the NICU setting

For Healthcare Professionals

Effectiveness and Feasibility of a Mindful Leadership Course for Medical Specialists: A Pilot Study [4]

This study evaluated the impact of a Mindful Leadership course on burnout, well-being, and leadership skills of medical specialists. Conducted from September 2014 to June 2016, it involved 52 medical specialists, with 48 completing the course. Results showed reductions in depersonalization, worry, and negative work-home interference, and improvements in mindfulness, life satisfaction, and self-reported ethical leadership. The course was found feasible with high completion rates, despite challenges in finding time to participate. This indicates the potential of such courses in ongoing professional development for medical specialists.

A Mindfulness Program to Improve Resident Physicians' Well-Being [5]

This study focuses on the feasibility and effectiveness of an 8-week mindfulness program designed to enhance the personal and work-related well-being of resident physicians. The program was tested with nine resident physicians at a major hospital in southern Germany. The study's methodology included evaluating changes in hair cortisol (a biomarker of stress) and self-reported personal and work-related well-being, using a pre-post within-subjects design.

The results indicated that the program was feasible in all assessed domains. Participants reported high satisfaction with the program, noting its helpfulness and personal and professional benefits. There was no study attrition, attendance was high, and participants engaged in an average of 13.5 min of daily home practice. The study observed a medium reduction in hair cortisol secretion and improvements in personal well-being indicators, such as perceived stress, mental health, self-attributed mindfulness, and self-compassion. Work-related well-being also improved, including reductions in job strain and work-related burnout and enhancements in thriving at work and physician empathy.

These findings suggest that the tailored mindfulness program is not only feasible but may also effectively reduce stress and improve both personal and work-related well-being among resident physicians. The positive outcomes of this study support further exploration through a randomized controlled trial to validate these preliminary results.

Mindfulness Meditation for Medical Students: A Student-Led Initiative to Expose Medical Students to Mindfulness Practices [6]

This study investigated the feasibility and impact of mindfulness training for medical students. Forty-one students were randomized into two groups: one receiving only an introductory mindfulness class and the other receiving this class plus an 8-week mindfulness meditation course. The findings indicated that mindfulness and awareness were inversely related to stress and depression. Students completing the full course showed greater familiarity and willingness to use mindfulness methods. However, there was no significant difference in wellness outcomes between the two groups. The study concluded that a mindfulness course is feasible for medical students and could be beneficial as a wellness and educational initiative. It also highlighted student aspirations for integrating mindfulness into medicine and medical education, despite recognizing the challenges involved.

Comparing the Effectiveness of Virtual and In-Person Delivery of Mindfulness-Based Skills Within Healthcare Curriculums [7]

This study explored the integration of mindfulness-based skills into physician assistant (PA) programs to promote well-being, especially considering the shift to virtual delivery due to pandemic restrictions. Over 2 years, first-year students in six PA programs participated in a mindfulness curriculum, with the first year being in-person and the second year virtual, while two other programs served as controls. The curriculum's effectiveness was assessed through surveys measuring mindfulness attributes (like decentering ability and present-moment awareness) and well-being factors (such as perceived stress and life satisfaction). Results indicated that the mindfulness curriculum was successful in enhancing mindfulness and life satisfaction, and reducing perceived stress, particularly when delivered in-person. Virtual delivery was also effective in reducing perceived stress but less so in improving life satisfaction. The study concluded that mindfulness-based skills, whether taught in-person or virtually, can effectively promote well-being in PA programs.

The Efficacy of Mindful Practice in Improving Diagnosis in Healthcare: A Systematic Review and Evidence Synthesis [8]

This study analyzed the role of mindful practice in enhancing clinical diagnosis accuracy. It reviewed a wide range of reports but found no randomized controlled trials on the subject. The majority of the evidence was based on conceptual commentary or opinion, with a small portion being controlled studies or comparative studies. While the findings suggest that mindful practice could be promising in improving diagnostic accuracy, definitive studies are needed to confirm this. The study also identified a taxonomy of terms related to mindful practice, highlighting seven core terms frequently used, which could focus future research for more generalizable findings.

References

1. Cengiz HÖ, et al. Effect of MINDFULNESS-based therapy on spiritual well-being in breast cancer patients: A randomized controlled study. Supportive Care in Cancer. 2023;31(7):438. https://doi.org/10.1007/s00520-023-07904-2. Accessed 27 Sept 2023.
2. Salajegheh Z, et al. Mindfulness-based stress reduction (MBSR) effects on the worries of women with poly cystic ovary syndrome (PCOS). BMC Psychiatry. 2023;23(1):185. https://doi.org/10.1186/s12888-023-04671-6.
3. Ginsberg KH, et al. Mindfulness and relaxation-based interventions to reduce parental stress, anxiety and/or depressive symptoms in the neonatal intensive care unit: A systematic review. J Clin Psychol Med Sett. 2023;30(2):387–402. https://doi.org/10.1007/s10880-022-09902-8.
4. Kersemaekers WM, et al. Effectiveness and feasibility of a mindful leadership course for medical specialists: A pilot study. BMC Med Educ. 2020;20(1):34. https://doi.org/10.1186/s12909-020-1948-5.

5. Fendel JC, et al. A mindfulness program to improve resident physicians' personal and work-related well-being: A feasibility study. Mindfulness. 2020;11(6):1511–9. https://doi.org/10.1007/s12671-020-01366-x. Accessed 11 Nov 2020.
6. Shapiro P, et al. Mindfulness meditation for medical students: A student-led initiative to expose medical students to mindfulness practices. Med Sci Educ. 2019;29(2):439–51. https://doi.org/10.1007/s40670-019-00708-2.
7. Hoover EB, et al. Comparing the effectiveness of virtual and in-person delivery of mindfulness-based skills within healthcare curriculums. Med Sci Educ. 2022;32(3):627–40. https://doi.org/10.1007/s40670-022-01554-5.
8. Pinnock R, et al. The efficacy of mindful practice in improving diagnosis in healthcare: A systematic review and evidence synthesis. Adv Health Sci Educ. 2021;26(3):785–809. https://doi.org/10.1007/s10459-020-10022-x.

Appendix C

Case Study: Exploring the Effectiveness of Mindfulness and Decentering Training in a Physician Assistant Curriculum

Eve B. Hoover and Bhupin Butaney

Given the rising epidemic of burnout among members of the healthcare team and the characteristically high-stress environment of health professions education, the authors saw a need to prioritize wellness principles within the classroom. Almost a decade of collaboration has led to a greater understanding of the variety of ways faculty can effectively deliver stress management tools to medical learners early on in education and training to foster professional resilience [1–5].

Together, they designed and implemented a method to incorporate mindfulness and decentering skills training into an existing course curriculum for first-year physician assistant (PA) students. After incorporating this curricular innovation, the feedback was so positive from students that we decided to study the curricular intervention formally so we might learn more about the current stress reduction practices incoming students were utilizing and to demonstrate how the addition of mindfulness and decentering training could improve life satisfaction, reduce perceived stress, and increase psychological flexibility.

We discovered a strong openness to mindfulness practices and an excellent opportunity with only 30% of students reporting prior experience with formal mindfulness-based practice. After presenting our initial findings to the professional community, the findings were so well received that several programs inquired about the intervention and how to partner with this study. The program to date has been incorporated into over 20 geographically diverse, public and private, PA education programs, and the findings strongly support inclusion of mindfulness skills training within wellness programs.

The 5-session curricula include many of the elements of the traditional Mindfulness-Based Stress Reduction (MBSR) techniques such as mindful breathing, mindful eating, awareness of pleasant and unpleasant sensations, beginner's mind, the power of perspective, and self-compassion, but was adapted for in-class lecture modules and out-of-class exercises with opportunities for formal self-reflection and instructor feedback [1, 6]. The curriculum also utilizes empirical literature, within a unique psychoeducation module, to bring relevancy to the medical learner on the causes for and impact of clinician burnout, the need for multilevel strategies including systemic, organizational, and individual approaches to support professional resiliency [1, 7].

As the multisite curriculum was occurring annually, we had an unexpected event create a tremendous opportunity to further test the merit of our intervention and to investigate the monumental impact of COVID-19 to student well-being. Given the requirement of virtual curricular delivery of all course content, including the mindfulness components of the curriculum, during the acute phase of COVID-19 pandemic, the authors also identified a unique opportunity to investigate the impact of the different delivery methods on learning outcomes. We aimed to address two central questions related to the training and education of healthcare providers: (1) Can mindfulness-based strategies designed to improve well-being and protect against stress encountered in PA education be effectively incorporated into course curriculum? (2) Can such a mindfulness-based curriculum be modified and delivered effectively using a virtual delivery format?

Over a 2-year period, we were able to assess incoming students starting their PA programs pre-pandemic (2019) and during the acute phase of the pandemic (2020). Six PA programs incorporated a mindfulness-based curriculum and two PA programs served as controls. Pre-pandemic the curriculum was delivered in person; during the acute-pandemic, the curriculum was delivered virtually. The in-person mindfulness curriculum was effective in increasing level of mindfulness, while decreasing perceived stress and improving life satisfaction when compared to the control. Similarly, when mindfulness curriculum was delivered virtually, students also reported increased levels of mindfulness and decreased levels of perceived stress.

When comparing pre- and acute-pandemic cohorts, we discovered that pre-pandemic participants reported significantly greater increases in perceived stress and decreases in life satisfaction compared to the acute-pandemic participants. These findings suggest that the impact on the pandemic student learner was on the whole supportive in terms of stress and life satisfaction. Our findings suggest that it is not only possible to incorporate mindfulness curricula within a course, but also this could be done through a virtual curriculum as well. Both learning delivery options were able to effectively increase mindfulness and life satisfaction, while mitigating increases in perceived stress. Levels of mindfulness increased in both years (pre-pandemic: 48%–71%, acute-pandemic: 51–74%). A substantial portion of participants also reported increases in life satisfaction (pre-pandemic: 54%, acute-pandemic: 47%). Furthermore, study findings demonstrate no difference in the magnitude of change for participants who received the mindfulness curriculum virtually vs. in-person.

Our findings support opportunities for expanding and diversifying well-being curricular platforms within health education curricula. These efforts hold promise for developing skills essential for professional resilience. In doing so, we may be able to improve the health and well-being of students and reduce clinician burnout throughout the medical career. These efforts should also have a positive impact on patient outcomes. This knowledge provides educators flexibility to approach curricular design using technology-based platforms that are often welcomed by students who value quick, readily accessible, multimedia platforms.

This project was not without its challenges. Several obstacles emerged through the process that included: coordinating reliance agreements with each institution; deciding whether to allow flexibility within each program's delivery to accommodate for institution, instructor, and geographical variation in cultures; developing a system to keep student information de-identified yet be able to reliably connect pre-test post-test responses. Programs were welcome to make minor curricular revisions as needed to support variation of program culture while ensuring consistency with the primary learning objectives. Heterogeneity in curricular design was reduced by developing a master version of the mindfulness curriculum, incorporating curricular tutorials for all program sites, sending yearly updates of resources and materials, and biannual team meetings for discussion and debrief. Over the years, we have incorporated a number of different strategies for the purpose of survey data matching; however, the most preferred solution has been use of four questions within the demographic section of the survey that are unique to each participant (i.e., last two numbers of phone number, first two letters of mother's first name, first two letters of the city of birth, last two letters of middle name). The answers to these questions are used as a template to develop the de-identified code utilized by the statistician for survey data matching.

Another obstacle addressed prior to the start to this study but essential to the viability of the project relates to the challenge of convincing program faculty and administrators of the material value of well-being and mindfulness initiatives as priority in education and training. As our institution is a medical education university, the core culture is rooted in the basic sciences to support application and practice of health services. Although acknowledging the importance of well-being and the potential for mindfulness strategies for personal growth and development, viewing it as a priority on par with clinical skills and understanding of scientific knowledge as essential for becoming an effective practitioner posed a challenge for systematic change to accommodate these components into an already packed curriculum. Initially weaving well-being content into a *Health Professionalism* course and Professional Development meetings, which was under the instructor purview to define essential components of professionalism, provided justification and recognition for its value through student feedback and course evaluations. We presented empirical evidence from change scores to faculty and administrators within the College of Health Sciences as part of an internal research series sponsored by the college. This stimulated interest and has led to many departments requesting lectures within several other health professions programs such as veterinary medicine, biomedical science, and speech language pathology.

Tying initiatives to accreditation [8] and expanded recognition that academic institutions are key players for fostering well-being of the future healthcare workforce [9] may assist in advocating for space within a curriculum to incorporate innovative programs focused on well-being [10, 11]. Providing evidence that links clinician well-being to reduction in medical errors and improved patient-centered care and practice may also be useful in justifying interventions to traditional outcomes [12, 13]. Lastly, the prevailing culture of faultless performance breeds and reinforces maladaptive perfectionism and impostor phenomenon in student learners. This predisposes them to higher risks of stress, lowers their ability to learn and remain creative in their problem-solving with patients while on clinical rotations and beyond. Recognizing that younger individuals are more vulnerable to mental health concerns [14–16] and are more open to seeking support for mental health concerns, it makes business sense for academic institutions to provide services that align with consumer needs. At our institution, we became intimately involved due to our research and program development with university initiatives to address the growing difficulties of our students who struggled and potentially dropped out, required leaves of absence, or were not doing well for a host of reasons.

We are enthusiastically beginning the ninth year of the curriculum and research. We have expanded our focus on well-being to investigate how mindfulness abilities may impact underlying risk factors such as cognitive patterns associated with maladaptive perfectionism and impostor phenomenon as well as protective factors associated with a mindset of self-compassion. We have also begun looking at mediators such as tolerance of ambiguity.

References

1. Hoover EB, Butaney B, Stoehr JD. Exploring the effectiveness of mindfulness and decentering training in a physician assistant curriculum. J Physician Assist Educ Off J Physician Assist Educ Assoc. 2020;31(1):19–22.
2. Hoover EB, Butaney B, Bernard K, Coplan B, LeLacheur S, Straker H, et al. Comparing the effectiveness of virtual and in-person delivery of mindfulness-based skills within healthcare curriculums. Med Sci Educ. 2022;32(3):627–40.
3. Hoover EB, Butaney B, LeLacheur S, Straker H, Bernard K, Coplan B, et al. Wellness in physician assistant education: exploring mindfulness, well-being, and stress. J Physician Assist Educ Off J Physician Assist Educ Assoc. 2022;33(2):107–13.
4. Neary S, Ruggeri M, Roman C, Hoover E, Butaney B, Weller I. Foundational skill-building in a novel well-being curriculum. J Physician Assist Educ. 2023;34(3):224–30.
5. Neary S, Ruggeri M, Roman C, Hoover E, Butaney B, Weller I. The effect of a well-being curriculum on the mental health outcomes of first-year PA students. JAAPA. 2021;34(12):1–2.
6. Kabat-Zinn J. Full catastrophe living: using the wisdom of your body and mind to face stress, pain, and illness. New York, NY: Bantam Books; 2013.
7. Hoover EB, Bernard KS. Call to action. Physician Assist Clin. 2022;7(1):89–102.
8. Accreditation Review Commission on Education for the Physician Assistant, Inc. Accreditation Standards for Physician Assistant Education, Fifth Edition [Internet]. 2019 [cited 2024 Feb 5]. https://www.arc-pa.org/accreditation/standards-of-accreditation/.
9. National Plan for Healthcare Workforce Well-being [Internet]. National Academy of Medicine; 2022 [cited 2024 Feb 5]. https://nam.edu/initiatives/clinician-resilience-and-well-being/national-plan-for-health-workforce-well-being/.

10. Knight AP, Rea M, Allgood JA, Sciolla AF, Haywood A, Stephens MB, et al. Bringing needed change to medical student well-being: A call to expand accreditation requirements. Teach Learn Med. 2023;35(1):101–7.
11. Slavin SJ, Schindler DL, Chibnall JT. Medical student mental health 3.0: Improving student wellness through curricular changes. Acad Med. 2014;89(4):573–7.
12. Gajewski PD, Boden S, Freude G, Potter GG, Falkenstein M. Burnout is associated with changes in error and feedback processing. Biol Psychol. 2017;129:349–58.
13. Prins JT, van der Heijden FMMA, Hoekstra-Weebers JEHM, Bakker AB, van de Wiel HBM, Jacobs B, et al. Burnout, engagement and resident physicians' self-reported errors. Psychol Health Med. 2009;14(6):654–66.
14. Gibbons S, Trette-McLean T, Crandall A, Bingham JL, Garn CL, Cox JC. Undergraduate students survey their peers on mental health: Perspectives and strategies for improving college counseling center outreach. J Am Coll Health. 2019;67(6):580–91.
15. Ketchen Lipson S, Gaddis SM, Heinze J, Beck K, Eisenberg D. Variations in student mental health and treatment utilization across US colleges and universities. J Am Coll Health. 2015;63(6):388–96.
16. Lucero JE, Emerson AD, Bowser T, Koch B. Mental health risk among members of the millennial population cohort: a concern for public health. Am J Health Promot. 2021;35(2):266–70.

Appendix D

Integrating Mindfulness into Graduate Medical Education: A Strategic Framework

Mission Statement

In the spirit of Competency-Based Medical Education (CBME), this document heralds a paradigm shift toward the inclusion of mindfulness as a cornerstone of graduate medical training, emphasizing its crucial role in fostering a well-rounded physician as is supported by modern science and cultural trends. This initiative supports the development of specific mindfulness-related competencies, such as attentional control and emotional regulation, through ongoing, longitudinal assessment and feedback. By doing so, we champion an adaptive educational model that not only respects but also capitalizes on the diversity of learning speeds and needs among residents.

Our mission, therefore, is to cultivate a new cadre of medical professionals who are as proficient in the application of mindfulness as they are in their clinical skills. We are committed to nurturing residents' personal growth and mastery of mindfulness practices, ensuring these skills are honed with the same precision and care as traditional medical competencies. In this transformative journey, continuous monitoring, assessment and feedback through new-age digital services serve as our compass and wand, guiding the integration of mindfulness in a manner that is both reflective and responsive to the evolving landscape of healthcare. Through this document, we lay out a strategic framework that positions mindfulness at the forefront of medical education.

Strategic Plan for Integrating Mindfulness Competencies into Medical Education

Articulating Outcome Competencies

We define the fabric of a competent medical professional not just by clinical acumen but also by the key, long unmeasurable traits of being a physician: attention, empathy, and compassion. Defined, existing competencies—attentional control to maintain presence in the moment, inhibition control to maintain composure under stress, emotional control to navigate the tumultuous seas of patient care, and behavioral control to exhibit professionalism—are the cardinal directions in which we can mindfully mold our residents. These competencies are real benchmarks against which we measure the transformation of medical students into mindful medical practitioners with equanimity.

Sequencing Competencies Progressively

Our educational blueprint lays a foundation with basic mindfulness awareness, ascending through the scaffolding of skill acquisition to the pinnacle of clinical integration. This journey commences with rudimentary techniques of breath work and progresses to the integration of mindfulness into the complex decision-making processes of medical practice. Each step is a building block in constructing a resilient physician, fortified against the rigors of healthcare delivery.

Facilitating Learning Experiences

Learning to be mindful is to immerse oneself in the art of experience. An ideal curriculum is a crucible where theory meets practice, from the quiet introspection of guided meditations to the dynamic application of mindfulness throughout the clinical workday. These experiences are not only meant to contribute to health maintenance but are also meant as strategic safeguards when a physician's character is tempered, ensuring they are not only sound in the mindset of medicine but also in the humanistic delivery of care.

- Structured Mindfulness Workshops: Incorporate regular workshops focusing on mindfulness techniques such as meditation, deep breathing exercises, and present-moment awareness.
- Clinical Application: Digitally integrate mindfulness practices into clinical rotations through app-based solutions, encouraging students to apply mindfulness in patient interactions, stressful procedures, and team dynamics.
- Mindful Reflection Sessions: Schedule regular reflective sessions where students can share experiences, challenges, and successes in applying mindfulness in their medical practice.

- Role-Play and Scenario-Based Training: Use role-play and simulated patient scenarios to both practice and demonstrate mindfulness skills, such as attentive control, empathetic listening and emotional regulation during patient interactions, or even instituting a physician-run group mindfulness session with patients and colleagues.
- Mindfulness Curriculum: Develop a formal, time-based curriculum of focused attention (FA) meditation that coincides with the learner's clinical mindfulness journey and that can be used to parallel benchmark milestones.
- Interprofessional Mindfulness Activities: Engage students in interprofessional activities that promote mindfulness across different healthcare disciplines, fostering a more holistic interdisciplinary approach to patient care.
- Incorporating Technology: Utilize digital platforms and apps for mindfulness training, allowing students to access mindfulness resources and exercises at their convenience, providing the key resource to monitor progress as well as institute research and track data.
- Mindfulness Mentoring Programs: Pair students with faculty or senior residents who are experienced in mindfulness practices for ongoing guidance and mentorship.
- Feedback and Evaluation: Include mindfulness as a component in performance evaluations and feedback, emphasizing its importance in the overall development of a medical professional.
- Continuous Learning Opportunities: Offer ongoing learning opportunities, such as seminars and guest lectures, on the latest research and techniques in mindfulness and its application in medicine.

Promoting Teaching Practices

Healthcare leaders are the architects of mindfulness in medicine, each a learner in their right. Faculty development programs are not merely adjuncts but rather essential cogs in our machinery. Ideal institutional leaders and faculty are those who are adept in the language of mindfulness, capable of imparting this wisdom in a manner that resonates with the individual learning cadences of our diverse resident population.

- Faculty Training in Mindfulness: Implement comprehensive training programs for faculty, focusing on mindfulness techniques and their integration into teaching. This training ensures that faculty members are not only familiar with mindfulness practices but can also effectively impart these skills.
- Incorporate Mindfulness into Teaching Methodologies: Encourage faculty to integrate mindfulness exercises into lectures, clinical teaching, and small group discussions. This could include starting classes with a brief mindfulness exercise to enhance focus or incorporating mindfulness-based case studies.
- Role Modeling by Faculty: Foster an environment where faculty members actively practice mindfulness themselves, serving as role models for students.

This practice demonstrates the practical application and benefits of mindfulness in a healthcare setting.
- Mindfulness-Based Communication Training: Provide special training for faculty on mindful communication, emphasizing listening, empathy, and presence in interactions with students and patients, providing a framework for sub-competency standard assessments during clinical rotations.
- Developing Mindful Learning Environments: Create learning spaces that promote mindfulness, such as quiet reflection areas or designated meditation spaces within the medical school or hospital.
- Interactive and Experiential Learning: Utilize interactive teaching methods that engage students in experiential learning of mindfulness, such as guided group meditations, mindful walking exercises, or reflective journaling sessions.
- Collaborative Teaching Approaches: Encourage collaborative teaching approaches where faculty and students across institutions share experiences and insights related to their home mindfulness practices, fostering a shared, digital learning environment.
- Faculty Observation and Feedback: Train faculty to observe and provide feedback on residents' application of mindfulness in clinical settings. This feedback should focus on areas like the resident's ability to remain present, maintain emotional balance, and demonstrate empathetic communication.
- Peer Teaching Opportunities: Facilitate peer teaching opportunities where senior students or residents can teach mindfulness techniques to their juniors, under faculty supervision. This approach not only reinforces the learners' skills but also enhances their teaching abilities.
- Regular Mindfulness Workshops for Faculty: Organize regular workshops and retreats dedicated to mindfulness for faculty, ensuring ongoing development and deepening of their mindfulness practice and teaching skills.

Supportive Assessment Practices

To assess mindfulness development alongside clinical competence, and moreover to try and develop positive associations between them, will require finely tuned coordination of self-report measures, as well as the development of an institutional framework for faculty and peer-to-peer monitoring and assessment. Importantly, currently existing clinical competency assessments, for instance, during Objective Structured Clinical Examinations (OSCEs), should be adapted to include mindfulness elements, such as scenarios that specifically evaluate a resident's ability to apply mindfulness in patient interactions or high-stress situations. The depth of a resident's independent mindfulness practice and self-reflection, including self-report measures, can be captured via digital applications.

Individualized Learning Trajectories

Recognizing the unique differences of each learner's mind, we eschew the one-size-fits-all approach. Our pedagogy is a mosaic of individualized learning experiences, from personalized digital learning platforms to the sage wisdom imparted in one-on-one coaching sessions. We empower our residents to chart their own course through the curriculum.

Systematic Approach to Learner Progression

The progression of a resident through the mindfulness competencies is an odyssey—a journey marked not by milestones but by a continuous thread of development. We employ a systematic, iterative approach to track this progression, using performance metrics and feedback loops that not only indicate where a resident is but also illuminate the path forward.

Inclusion of Mindfulness in Medical Training

The evolving landscape of medical education now incorporates mindfulness training, responding to societal needs and advancing the medical profession's values. This inclusion aims to develop physicians who are technically skilled and emotionally intelligent, capable of empathetic and composed patient care.

Our outcome-based educational approach focuses on developing the core attributes of a mindful physician, emphasizing compassion, well-being, and improved patient care. Mindfulness is integrated as a vital skill in various aspects of medical practice, enhancing focus and reducing stress. This integration extends to Entrustable Professional Activities (EPAs), ensuring mindfulness is a key component of clinical responsibility.

The training emphasizes deep learning, moving beyond basic understanding to deeply ingrained mindfulness practices. Residents engage in practical applications of these skills, learning through real-world experiences. Mindfulness is positioned as a fundamental aspect of their professional identity, built on self-care and resilience.

Our educational strategy employs the Zone of Proximal Development, challenging residents to grow their mindfulness skills. Personalized coaching and continuous learning are central to this learner-centered approach. Assessments, both programmatic and formative, track residents' progress, providing feedback that guides their mindfulness journey.

Learning analytics play a crucial role in evaluating the impact of mindfulness training, shaping our approach to meet each resident's needs. Our goal is to cultivate a new generation of physicians proficient in mindfulness, thereby enriching the medical field and enhancing patient care.

Anticipating and Addressing Challenges in Mindfulness Integration

As we embark on this transformative journey to integrate mindfulness into CBME, we must navigate potential challenges with foresight and agility.

Defining Mindfulness Competencies

In the quest to define mindfulness competencies, clarity is paramount. Yet, the intangible nature of mindfulness may cast shadows of ambiguity on our path. To transcend this, we will craft competencies with precision, ensuring they resonate with the clinical reality and mirror the inner landscape of mindful practice. We are mindful that these competencies must be as palpable and assessable as any clinical skill.

Performance Benchmarks and Milestones

The establishment of performance benchmarks and milestones for mindfulness may be met with the challenge of quantifying the qualitative. The nuanced subtleties of mindfulness practices defy simple measurement. We will rise to this challenge by sculpting benchmarks that are both measurable and meaningful, capturing the essence of mindfulness in the crucible of clinical competence.

Competency Assessment

The implementation of a new competency assessment or standard for mindfulness ventures into uncharted territories and is not the aim of our framework. It is important to note that our milestone competency is based on the coordinated, routine procurement of validated self-report measures, as well as tailored clinical skills and clerkship evaluations.

Stakeholder Engagement and Buy-In

Engaging stakeholders and fostering buy-in is akin to nurturing a garden of diverse flora. Each stakeholder brings a different perspective, which may sometimes clash with the collective vision. Through dialogue, demonstration, and dedication, we will cultivate a shared understanding and appreciation for the value mindfulness brings to medical practice.

- Hosting Collaborative Workshops: Organize workshops where stakeholders, including faculty, residents, healthcare administrators, and students, can discuss the role and benefits of mindfulness in medical practice. Use these sessions for open dialogue and exchange of ideas.

Appendix D

- Demonstration Sessions: Conduct demonstration sessions where the effects and techniques of mindfulness are showcased, providing stakeholders with firsthand experience of its benefits.
- Regular Meetings with Stakeholders: Establish regular meetings with different stakeholder groups to discuss the integration of mindfulness into the curriculum and clinical practice. These meetings can serve to address concerns, gather suggestions, and keep everyone informed about the progress and impact of mindfulness initiatives.
- Incorporating Feedback Mechanisms: Create channels for stakeholders to provide ongoing feedback about mindfulness programs. This could include surveys, suggestion boxes, or digital platforms.
- Engaging Leadership: Involve institutional leaders in promoting mindfulness initiatives. Their endorsement and participation can significantly enhance buy-in across all levels of the institution.
- Pilot Programs: Launch pilot mindfulness programs in certain departments or units. The success and learnings from these pilots can be used to demonstrate the value of mindfulness to the wider institution.
- Reporting Outcomes and Success Stories: Share success stories and data on the positive outcomes of mindfulness practices, such as reduced burnout rates or improved patient care, to reinforce its value.
- Peer Champions: Identify and empower "mindfulness champions" within various stakeholder groups who can advocate for mindfulness practices among their peers.
- Integrating into Existing Programs: Seamlessly integrate mindfulness training into existing educational and clinical programs, making it a natural part of the medical training environment.
- Ongoing Education and Resources: Provide accessible resources and ongoing educational opportunities related to mindfulness for all stakeholders, ensuring they have the knowledge and tools to effectively engage with and support mindfulness practices.

Regular Evaluation and Feedback

Instituting a regular cadence of evaluation and feedback will require a cultural shift. The rhythm of medical training is fast-paced, often leaving little room for reflection. We will introduce feedback mechanisms that are both efficient and effective, integrating seamlessly into the existing workflow, thereby maintaining the harmony of the educational symphony.

- Integration into Existing Review Processes: Align mindfulness evaluation with the existing review and assessment processes for clinical competencies. This integration ensures mindfulness is seen as a fundamental component of medical training.

- Scheduled Feedback Sessions: Set up regular, structured feedback sessions between faculty and residents. These could be weekly or bi-weekly and focus on discussing residents' progress, challenges, and areas for improvement.
- Real-Time Feedback in Clinical Settings: Encourage faculty to provide immediate, on-the-spot feedback during clinical rotations, promoting application of mindfulness techniques in real time.
- Use of Digital Platforms for Continuous Teaching and Feedback: Implement digital platforms where faculty can regularly record and share feedback with residents and faculty across multiple institutions. These platforms can also allow residents to ask questions and seek advice from experienced teachers outside of their independent practice.
- Faculty Development for Effective Feedback: Train faculty members on how to provide effective, constructive feedback, especially in the context of mindfulness. This training ensures that feedback is not only informative but also supports the resident's growth.
- Feedback-Focused Workshops or Seminars: Organize workshops or seminars specifically aimed at improving feedback techniques. These could include role-playing exercises and peer-review sessions.
- Documentation and Follow-up: Ensure all feedback is documented and followed up in subsequent sessions. This approach helps track progress over time and reinforces the importance of continuous development.

Long-Term Engagement and Adaptation

Acknowledging that the integration of mindfulness, let alone the development of mindfulness trait itself, is a marathon, not a sprint, we foresee the challenge of sustaining momentum over time. Our commitment to long-term engagement will ensure that mindfulness remains a vibrant thread woven through the tapestry of medical education.

- Long-Term Research and Evaluation: Conduct long-term studies and evaluations to assess the impact of mindfulness training on students' performance, well-being, and patient care are the cornerstone to this program. Findings can be used for essential mindfulness research but also to adapt and refine the mindfulness curriculum.
- Promoting a Mindful Institutional Culture: Work toward creating a culture that values and practices mindfulness at all levels, from administrative staff to clinical faculty and students.
- Adapting to Changing Needs and Feedback: Stay responsive to the changing needs of students and faculty regarding mindfulness training and adapt the program accordingly. This could involve updating training methods, incorporating new mindfulness techniques, and addressing specific challenges faced by the community.

Appendix D

Harmonizing Competencies

The harmonization of mindfulness competencies with existing frameworks presents a complex puzzle, though their inclusion is not forced and complements, rather than overshadows, the existing ACGME milestone framework and medical curriculum.

- Mapping Mindfulness to Clinical Skills: Through research, identify and map specific aspects of mindfulness that contribute to the development of clinical skills, such as improved focus in patient care or enhanced communication skills.
- Incorporating into Evaluation Tools: Modify existing evaluation and assessment tools to include mindfulness elements. For example, adding mindfulness-related criteria to OSCEs or 360° evaluations.
- Creating Cross-Disciplinary Mindfulness Modules: Develop cross-disciplinary modules or workshops that incorporate mindfulness training, showing its relevance across various medical specialties.
- Regular Curriculum Review and Adaptation: Establish a regular review process to ensure the mindfulness competencies remain relevant and effectively integrated within the evolving medical education landscape.
- Feedback from Medical Community: Gather and incorporate feedback from students, faculty, and healthcare professionals on the integration of mindfulness into the curriculum, ensuring it meets the needs and expectations of the medical community.
- Pilot Programs and Iterative Implementation: Implement pilot programs to test the integration of mindfulness competencies in certain areas of the curriculum, using feedback and results to refine and expand the integration.
- Documentation and Resource Development: Develop comprehensive documentation and resources that clearly outline how mindfulness competencies are integrated into the ACGME milestones, providing clarity and guidance for educators and students.

Accreditation Models

Finally, integrating mindfulness competencies into accreditation models may test the traditional boundaries of regulatory structures. We approach this not as a barrier, but as an opportunity to expand the horizons of accreditation, advocating for models that recognize the full spectrum of physician competencies.

Practical Integration of Mindfulness into the Existing Milestone Framework

Developing Mindfulness-Related Milestones

Within the established Milestone framework, we introduce a novel tier: mindfulness-related competencies. Each level delineates the progression from novice, where a student or resident begins to cultivate awareness of the present moment, to expert, where they not only apply mindfulness in complex clinical situations but also guide others. For example, at the novice level, a resident may learn to employ basic breathing techniques to maintain focus during patient interactions. As they progress, they would demonstrate increased ability to manage stress in high-acuity settings and eventually lead team-based mindfulness sessions, promoting a calm, focused, and empathic approach to patient care.

Criterion-Based Assessment

Mindfulness competencies are assessed with a keen eye on the individual's actual performance in real-world scenarios. For instance, a resident's ability to maintain composure and patient engagement, as can be assessed by use of a digital meditation session or calming exercise during a difficult work scenario or even during downtime, the use of app-based, guided group meditations with team members or patients, or even observed, documented mindful behavior by peers and faculty (as recorded in student and resident evaluations) during a stressful on-call night would be a benchmark for assessing emotional regulation. These assessments are structured to reflect the residents' personal growth trajectory, irrespective of their year in the program, ensuring that each learner's journey toward mindfulness is measured against clear, objective criteria.

Observable Behaviors and Attributes

To bring the abstract concept of mindfulness into the concrete realm of assessment, we pinpoint observable behaviors. A resident may be evaluated on their ability to remain attentive throughout patient interactions, demonstrate empathetic communication, and utilize mindfulness techniques to mitigate burnout. These behaviors are documented and reviewed, providing tangible evidence of the resident's development in mindfulness. The following clinical scenarios provide an example of how such observable behaviors and attributes can be documented and reviewed;

- Clinical Scenario 1: High-Stress Emergency Room Setting
  - Observable Behavior: A resident utilizes a 15-min break dedicated to body scan or breath work to maintain calm and focus after managing a string of emergency cases.
  - Attributes Evaluated: Ability to apply mindfulness techniques to stay centered and make ongoing clear decisions under fatigue and pressure.
- Clinical Scenario 2: Difficult Patient Interaction
  - Observable Behavior: During an interaction with a non-compliant or aggressive patient, the resident demonstrates patience, active listening, and empathetic communication or chooses to employ a joint mindfulness exercise with the patient.

Appendix D

- Attributes Evaluated: Use of mindfulness to understand patient perspectives and respond with empathy and support, rather than react impulsively.

- Clinical Scenario 3: Long Surgical Procedure
  - Observable Behavior: The resident communicates the active use of breath monitoring to anchor themselves to the steps of the surgery.
  - Attributes Evaluated: Sustained attention and focus, indicative of regular mindfulness practice.

- Clinical Scenario 4: End-of-Life Care Discussion
  - Observable Behavior: In discussions about end-of-life care, the resident shows compassionate communication, balancing clinical information with empathy.
  - Attributes Evaluated: Mindfulness in maintaining emotional balance and providing patient-centered care.

- Clinical Scenario 5: Peer-to-Peer Interaction
  - Observable Behavior: The resident actively supports and collaborates with peers during challenging clinical situations, specifically employing or teaching mindfulness techniques.
  - Attributes Evaluated: Application of mindfulness in interpersonal skills and teamwork.

- Clinical Scenario 6: Personal Reflection and Self-Care
  - Observable Behavior: The resident engages in self-care practices and digitally recorded reflective exercises, contributing to discussions about personal and professional development.
  - Attributes Evaluated: Self-awareness and commitment to personal mindfulness practice as part of professional growth.

- Clinical Scenario 7: Feedback Reception
  - Observable Behavior: When receiving critical feedback, the resident listens attentively, reflects thoughtfully, and responds constructively, possibly choosing to enter or exit the critical feedback with a brief mindfulness.
  - Attributes Evaluated: Mindful reception of feedback, demonstrating openness and a growth mindset.

Guiding Curriculum Development

Once implemented, the mindfulness milestones will illuminate the path for ongoing curriculum development, highlighting areas ripe for integration of mindfulness training. For instance, prior to rotations traditionally heavy in technical skill acquisition, additional modules can be assigned to instill regular, daily adoption of inner awareness and stress management techniques.

Formative Purpose

In service of a formative purpose, mindfulness milestones offer a reflective mirror for residents. They are tools for self-assessment and program improvement, not punitive measures. These milestones serve as a compass, helping residents navigate their internal landscape as diligently as they do the complexities of patient care.

Complementing Other Assessments

Mindfulness milestones enhance, not replace, the existing array of assessments. They offer a new dimension, providing insights into the residents' holistic development, including their interpersonal dynamics, emotional intelligence, and resilience. These competencies are woven into the larger fabric of medical training assessments, ensuring a comprehensive evaluation of the residents' capabilities.

Frequent Revisions and Updates

As the field of mindfulness and its application in medicine evolves, so too will our milestones. We commit to the regular re-evaluation and updating of these benchmarks, ensuring they remain at the forefront of educational best practices and reflect the latest in mindfulness research and clinical application.

Stakeholder Engagement and Feedback

Incorporating mindfulness into medical training is a collaborative effort, drawing on the insights and experiences of all stakeholders. Through regular feedback sessions, the milestones are refined, and their practical application is honed. Residents, faculty, and other healthcare professionals contribute their perspectives, ensuring the milestones for mindfulness resonate with the realities of medical practice with respect to each individual institution.

Avoiding Overemphasis on Short Rotations

While short rotations offer a snapshot of clinical skill, mindfulness development is a longer arc. We caution against an overreliance on brief assessments for mindfulness competencies. Instead, we track the residents' growth in mindfulness over their entire clinical education, ideally starting during medical school, offering a more accurate reflection of their internalization and application of these practices.

Appendix D

Faculty Involvement in Mindfulness Integration

Familiarization with Mindfulness Milestones

The vanguard of this mindfulness initiative is our faculty, whose expertise and guidance are pivotal. We embark on an educational campaign to ensure all faculty members are well-versed in the structure and purpose of the newly integrated mindfulness milestones. This familiarization transcends disciplinary boundaries, involving not just physicians but all interprofessional team members. Faculty members are encouraged to delve into the mindfulness subcompetencies themselves, aligning their understanding with the overarching goals of these milestones.

Focusing on Relevant Subcompetencies and Milestones

Faculty engagement is further refined by aligning their specific roles and educational settings with relevant mindfulness subcompetencies. Evaluation forms and teaching materials are tailored, weaving mindfulness into the fabric of everyday clinical education. This approach allows faculty to authentically integrate mindfulness principles into their teaching, making it a natural extension of their existing expertise.

Faculty Development in Assessment and Feedback

To reinforce this integration, we initiate comprehensive faculty development programs. These sessions, workshops, and seminars concentrate on enhancing faculty's ability to assess and provide feedback on mindfulness competencies. Special emphasis is placed on direct observation techniques, enabling faculty to identify and reinforce mindfulness-related behaviors and attitudes in clinical settings.

Commitment to Refining Assessment Skills

Continuous improvement is the cornerstone of our approach. Faculty are encouraged to engage in an ongoing process of refining their assessment skills, specifically in relation to mindfulness. Resources, regular workshops, and peer-learning opportunities are made available, fostering an environment of continual professional growth and learning.

Feedback to Improve Assessment Approaches

Faculty members are not just educators but also collaborators in this initiative. Their feedback is instrumental in shaping and improving the mindfulness assessment approaches. We establish channels for open, constructive communication, allowing faculty to share their insights and experiences, which in turn inform the evolution of our mindfulness assessment strategies.

Meaningful Narrative Assessment

In assessing mindfulness, the power of narrative is unparalleled. Faculty are guided to provide meaningful narrative assessments, capturing the nuances of a resident's mindfulness practice. These narratives serve as valuable tools for program directors and Clinical Competency Committees, offering a depth of insight that complements quantitative measures.

Ongoing Feedback for Learners

The faculty's role in providing continuous, actionable feedback to learners is underscored. This feedback is a crucial mechanism through which residents can gauge their progress in developing mindfulness competencies, receiving both encouragement and constructive critique.

Supporting Faculty in Mindfulness Integration

To support this paradigm shift, we provide faculty with the necessary resources and tools to seamlessly integrate mindfulness into their teaching and assessment practices. This includes access to mindfulness training resources, teaching aids, and a supportive community that values and practices mindfulness. We foster a culture where mindfulness is not only taught but also embodied by our faculty, making it a living, breathing aspect of our educational ethos.

Assessment of Mindfulness in Core Competencies

Patient Care

- Direct Observation: In the clinical settings, our evaluators will observe how residents employ mindfulness during patient interactions. The focus will be on their ability to remain present, manage stress effectively, initiate individual or group mindful exercises, and maintain patient-centered care even in high-pressure situations.
- Simulation with Standardized Patients: By introducing scenarios that challenge the residents' mindfulness skills, such as managing difficult conversations or navigating emotionally charged clinical situations, we assess their ability to apply mindfulness techniques in real time. This simulation acts as a rehearsal stage for honing the art of mindful patient care.

Appendix D

Medical Knowledge

- Direct Observation and Oral Questioning: Evaluators will assess residents' understanding of mindfulness principles through direct questioning during clinical rounds, looking for insights into how mindfulness techniques helped inform their medical reasoning and decision-making.
- In-Training Examinations: Examination papers will integrate cases and questions that probe the residents' overall understanding of mindfulness and its individual components.

Professionalism

- Multi-Source Feedback and Patient Surveys: Feedback from peers, faculty, and patients will provide a panoramic view of the residents' professionalism, particularly their empathetic engagement, resilience in the face of challenges, and emotional regulation—all hallmarks of a mindful practitioner.
- Direct Observation: Observations will focus on residents' demeanor and implementation of mindfulness techniques in various situations, assessing their ability to maintain professionalism imbued with mindfulness, especially in handling ethical dilemmas and stressful scenarios.

Interpersonal and Communication Skills

- Multi-Source Feedback and Patient Surveys: These assessments will gauge how mindfulness enhances residents' communication skills, looking at their ability to engage in active listening and empathetic interaction with patients, families, and team members.
- Simulation with Standardized Patients: Simulated interactions will test and observe the residents' application of mindfulness in their communication, assessing their capacity to maintain patient-centered and compassionate dialogues.

Practice-Based Learning and Improvement

- Reflective Practice Rubrics: Residents will engage in reflective practices, guided by rubrics that evaluate their ability to introspect and apply mindfulness in their learning and clinical practice.
- Evidence-Based Medicine Logs: These logs will include key, qualitative reflections on how mindfulness influences their overall competency and clinical decisions, as well as impacts patient outcomes, integrating mindfulness into the fabric of evidence-based practice.

Systems-Based Practice

- Quality Improvement Knowledge Assessment: This assessment will evaluate how residents' mindfulness practice contributes to system-level improvements, like enhancing teamwork efficiency and reducing clinician burnout.
- Multi-Source Feedback: Feedback from various sources will provide insights into how residents integrate mindfulness into their approach to systems-based practice, influencing healthcare delivery and team dynamics.

Benefits of Mindfulness Integration

- Enhanced Feedback: The integration of mindfulness into milestones equips educators with a robust tool for providing nuanced feedback, fostering both professional expertise and personal growth among residents.
- A New Assessment Language: Mindfulness competencies introduce a fresh lexicon for assessment, bridging gaps in understanding and fostering a unified perspective on these essential skills.
- Curricular Gap Identification: The mindfulness framework shines a light on previously overlooked areas in the curriculum, particularly those pertaining to emotional intelligence and stress management, paving the way for a more holistic medical education.
- Early Identification of Challenges: By embedding mindfulness competencies, educators can swiftly identify and address struggles in residents, particularly in managing stress and emotional responses.
- Faculty Development Opportunities: The mindfulness initiative necessitates and catalyzes faculty development, equipping educators with vital skills to teach and assess these new competencies.
- Continuous Quality Improvement: Mindfulness becomes a cornerstone in the continuous quality improvement of medical education, evolving and adapting as it is taught and assessed.
- Enriching Medical Education Research: The inclusion of mindfulness adds a rich, new dimension to medical education research, particularly in studies focusing on well-being and physician burnout.

Challenges and Solutions

- Time and Resource Constraints: We propose integrating mindfulness assessments into existing workflows, thereby minimizing additional burdens and enhancing efficiency.
- Synthesizing Assessments: Clear, structured guidelines will be developed for incorporating mindfulness assessments within the Clinical Competency Committee's developmental judgments.

Appendix D

- Assessment Tool Alignment: We aim to align existing assessment forms with mindfulness competencies to ensure a coherent and unified evaluation process.
- Development of Specific Assessment Methods: The creation and adaptation of mindfulness-specific assessment tools will address the current lack of tailored methods.
- Managing Cognitive Load: Mindfulness evaluations will be integrated into broader competency assessments, effectively balancing the cognitive load during rotations.
- Prioritizing Faculty Development: Faculty development programs will be designed with a focus on mindfulness competencies, ensuring educators are well-prepared to teach and evaluate these skills.
- Streamlining Faculty Assessment Processes: To reduce the assessment burden on faculty, we will streamline these processes, providing necessary support and resources.
- Overcoming Short Faculty Exposure: For shorter faculty attending periods, we will develop methods to assess mindfulness competencies that do not require prolonged exposure.
- Adapting to 1-Year Fellowships: The five-level milestone rubric will be adapted for shorter training programs, focusing on key mindfulness competencies.
- Simplifying Educational Jargon: Mindfulness concepts will be communicated in clear, accessible language, enhancing understanding among all stakeholders and avoiding overly complex educational jargon (Table D.1).

Mindful Learning in Medical Training: A Sample Path

- Incorporating Mindfulness in Early Stages:
  - Context: Beginning with preclinical years.
  - Method: Introductory lectures on mindfulness.
  - Impact: Builds foundational understanding and acceptance of mindfulness principles.
- Workshops and Longitudinal Programs:
  - Context: Throughout preclinical and clinical training.
  - Method: Regular workshops and longitudinal programs focusing on mindfulness meditation, stress reduction, and self-care using mindfulness techniques.
  - Impact: Equips students with ongoing tools to handle stress, enhance focus, and develop resilience.
- Curriculum Integration:
  - Context: Embedding mindfulness within existing courses.
  - Method: Role-playing exercises and simulated patient encounters in clinical skills courses.
  - Impact: Promotes mindful presence, empathy, and effective communication.

Table D.1 Assessment of mindfulness in core competencies

Competency	Level 1 (novice)	Level 2 (advanced beginner)	Level 3 (competent)	Level 4 (proficient)	Level 5 (expert)
Patient care: Mindful practice	Recognizes basic mindfulness techniques Begins to apply these in simple patient interactions under supervision	Demonstrates improved focus and presence during patient interactions Starts to apply stress management techniques	Independently integrates mindfulness in patient care, showing improved emotional regulation	Coaches junior residents in applying mindfulness in clinical settings Exhibits advanced empathy and patient engagement	Serves as a role model in mindful patient care. Leads mindfulness workshops or initiatives in clinical settings
Medical knowledge: Mindfulness application	Has basic understanding of the principles of mindfulness and its benefits in healthcare	Applies basic mindfulness principles to enhance clinical decision-making under guidance	Consistently applies mindfulness principles to improve clinical outcomes and personal well-being	Teaches and explains the application of mindfulness in complex clinical scenarios to peers	Develops innovative approaches to integrate mindfulness in medical practice and shares expertise widely
Professionalism: Mindful communication and ethics	Demonstrates basic respectful communication in clinical settings Beginning to understand the role of mindfulness in professional behavior	Shows improved communication skills, using mindfulness to manage stressful situations more effectively	Exhibits professionalism in challenging scenarios, using mindfulness to maintain ethical standards and composure	Serves as a mentor in guiding others on how to use mindfulness for professional growth	Recognized leader in advocating for ethical practice and mindful communication in the medical community
Interpersonal and communication skills: Mindful interactions	Learning to listen actively and communicate with mindfulness under supervision	Shows increased ability to engage patients and team members with a mindful approach	Skillfully uses mindful communication to enhance team dynamics and patient rapport	Coaches others in developing their mindful communication skills	Exemplifies and inspires excellence in mindful communication at an institutional level
Practice-based learning and improvement: Reflective mindfulness	Engages in basic reflective practices related to mindfulness and clinical experiences	Uses reflective practices to identify personal learning needs in mindfulness and clinical skills	Regularly uses reflection to improve personal mindfulness practice and patient care	Leads peer group reflections, facilitating learning and improvement in mindfulness	Pioneers advanced reflective practices, contributing significantly to the field of mindfulness in medicine
Systems-based practice: Mindfulness in healthcare systems	Recognizes the role of mindfulness in systems-based practice	Begins to apply mindfulness to navigate and improve healthcare systems	Effectively uses mindfulness to contribute to system improvements and team wellness	Leads initiatives that integrate mindfulness into systems-based practice	Recognized as a thought leader in applying mindfulness for systemic healthcare improvements

Appendix D   211

- Mindfulness in Study Routines:
  - Context: Independent study and revision times.
  - Method: Demonstrating mindfulness implementation into study breaks.
  - Impact: Improves concentration and reduces burnout during intensive study periods.
- Mindful Engagement in Classrooms:
  - Context: Anatomy, physiology, and pathology classes.
  - Method: Integrating mindfulness exercises to deepen understanding and foster emotional processing.
  - Impact: Enhances learning and cultivates a deeper appreciation of medical science.
- Access to Mindfulness Resources:
  - Context: Support outside the classroom.
  - Method: Providing free or discounted subscriptions to mindfulness apps and quiet spaces for meditation.
  - Impact: Facilitates continuous and independent practice of mindfulness.
- Faculty Engagement:
  - Context: Role of educators in promoting mindfulness.
  - Method: Encouraging faculty to integrate mindfulness in their teaching.
  - Impact: Creates a more holistic and empathetic learning environment.

Modern Medical School Curriculum with Integrated Mindfulness Training

Year 1: Building the Foundation

- Introduction to Medicine and Mindfulness:
  - Focus: Orientation to medical education and an introduction to mindfulness.
  - Method: Workshops and lectures on mindfulness basics, its science, and relevance in medicine.
  - Peer Influence: Senior students share experiences and benefits of mindfulness in their medical journey.
- Basic Sciences and Mindful Learning:
  - Subjects: Anatomy, Physiology, Biochemistry, etc.
  - Method: Start each class with a brief mindfulness exercise, like a body scan or focused breathing.
  - Application: Encourage mindful study habits and group discussions.

- Clinical Skills and Mindful Communication:
  - Focus: Introduction to patient interactions.
  - Method: Role-playing exercises with a focus on teaching mindful breathing, practicing mindful listening, and further exploring an understanding of empathy.
  - Peer Influence: Residents demonstrate mindful patient communication techniques.
- Mindfulness Practice Sessions:
  - Frequency: Weekly or bi-weekly.
  - Focus: Guided meditation, stress management, and reflective journaling.
  - Peer Influence: Facilitated by senior students, promoting community and support.

Year 2: Deepening Understanding and Application

- Pathophysiology and Mindful Observation:
  - Subjects: Pathology, Microbiology, Pharmacology, etc.
  - Method: Continue meditation exercises before class or laboratory work.
  - Application: Individual journal or group reflective practice on how mindfulness aids in understanding disease processes.
- Clinical Rotations Prep and Mindful Resilience:
  - Focus: Preparation for clinical rotations.
  - Method: Workshops on implementing mindfulness into the daily clinical schedule, as well as utilizing it rapidly and efficiently in response to a multitude of novel experiences which are to be had.
  - Peer Influence: Senior residents share experience and strategies for maintaining mindfulness during rotations.
- Mindful Peer Support Groups:
  - Focus: Sharing experiences and challenges.
  - Method: Regular group meetings containing trainees across all levels for discussion and support.
  - Peer Influence: Guided by senior students, fostering a culture of mindfulness.

Year 3: Clinical Rotations and Mindfulness in Practice

- Rotations in Various Specialties:
  - Focus: Hands-on patient care in different departments.

Appendix D

- Application: Mindfulness in patient interactions, stress management, and decision-making.
- Peer Influence: Clinical fellows and senior residents as continued role models for applying mindfulness in clinical settings.

• Mindfulness in Challenging Situations:
  - Focus: Managing difficult patient interactions or emotional cases.
  - Method: Debriefing sessions with mindfulness reflection on emotional responses.

• Advanced Mindfulness Workshops:
  - Focus: Deepening mindfulness skills among more experienced meditators (advanced, expert).
  - Method: Advanced meditation techniques, mindful leadership, and empathy exercises.

Year 4: Specialization and Mindful Leadership

• Electives and Research:
  - Focus: Pursuing areas of interest or research.
  - Application: Implementing mindfulness in research settings and specialty choices.

• Pre-Residency Training and Mindfulness Integration:
  - Focus: Transition to residency.
  - Method: Workshops on incorporating mindfulness into a resident's routine and leadership roles.
  - Peer Influence: Interaction with current residents who practice mindfulness.

• Mindful Mentorship Program:
  - Focus: Mentoring underclassmen.
  - Method: Senior students guide younger peers in mindfulness practices, continuing the cycle of learning and support.

Overall Curriculum Highlights

- Progressive development of mindfulness skills over 4 years.
- Regular integration of mindfulness in academic and clinical settings.
- Strong emphasis on peer support and mentorship to foster a community of mindful practitioners.

Opportunities for Faculty

Scenario 1: Faculty Introduction to Mindfulness

- Setting: Faculty development sessions at the start of the academic year.
- Focus: Introduce mindfulness principles, benefits in teaching, and stress management for faculty.
- Organizational Schematic: Mandated faculty training, inclusion in faculty development programs.
- Review: Feedback sessions in departmental meetings to discuss implementation and challenges.

Scenario 2: Mindful Teaching Methods

- Setting: Regular faculty meetings.
- Focus: Incorporating mindfulness into teaching strategies, such as starting lectures with mindfulness exercises.
- Organizational Schematic: Encourage faculty to share successful mindfulness practices in meetings.
- Review: Quarterly reviews of teaching methods, with mindfulness integration as a key metric.

Scenario 3: Mindfulness in Clinical Supervision

- Setting: Clinical settings with student rotations.
- Focus: Faculty demonstrating mindfulness in patient care and student interactions.
- Organizational Schematic: Integration of mindfulness practices in clinical teaching guidelines.
- Review: Regular assessments of clinical teaching effectiveness, including mindfulness aspects.

Scenario 4: Faculty-Led Student Mindfulness Workshops

- Setting: Workshops throughout the academic year.
- Focus: Faculty leading mindfulness workshops for students, focusing on stress reduction and empathy.
- Organizational Schematic: Workshops as part of the curriculum, led by trained faculty members.
- Review: Student feedback and workshop effectiveness analysis in curriculum review meetings.

Appendix D

Scenario 5: Research and Mindfulness

- Setting: Research methodology classes and seminars.
- Focus: Discussing the role of mindfulness in research, maintaining focus and ethical considerations.
- Organizational Schematic: Incorporation of mindfulness discussions in research training and meetings.
- Review: Evaluation of research training modules, including mindfulness content, during faculty meetings.

Scenario 6: Integrating Mindfulness in Problem-Based Learning

- Setting: Small group learning sessions.
- Focus: Faculty guiding students in mindful problem-solving and reflective practices.
- Organizational Schematic: Structured problem-based learning sessions with embedded mindfulness practices.
- Review: Analysis of problem-based learning effectiveness, with mindfulness as a component.

Scenario 7: Mindfulness in Exam Preparation

- Setting: Sessions prior to major examinations.
- Focus: Faculty teaching mindfulness techniques to manage exam stress and enhance concentration.
- Organizational Schematic: Scheduled mindfulness sessions during exam preparation periods and immediately prior to and following examinations.
- Review: Post-exam debriefs to gauge effectiveness of mindfulness in reducing exam stress.

Scenario 8: Faculty Peer Support Groups

- Setting: Regularly scheduled faculty meetings.
- Focus: Creating faculty mindfulness support groups for stress management and collegial support.
- Organizational Schematic: Establishment of mindfulness peer groups, supported by administration.
- Review: Regular check-ins at administrative meetings to assess group effectiveness and participation.

Scenario 9: Mindfulness in Faculty Evaluation and Feedback

- Setting: Faculty performance reviews.
- Focus: Including mindfulness as a criterion in teaching evaluations and peer reviews.
- Organizational Schematic: Modification of evaluation forms to include mindfulness aspects.
- Review: Annual reviews to assess faculty performance, including mindfulness practice and teaching.

Scenario 10: Integrating Mindfulness in High-Level Strategic Planning

- Setting: Executive board meetings and strategic planning sessions.
- Focus: Considering mindfulness as a strategic priority in overall educational goals and faculty development.
- Organizational Schematic: Mindfulness as a key component in strategic educational planning.
- Review: Annual high-level administrative meetings to review progress and set future goals related to mindfulness integration.

Appendix E

This appendix is meant to be utilized by healthcare teams to practice implementation of mindfulness techniques in group, mock settings. Use the scenarios to imagine overcoming potential hurdles related to burnout and DEI with mindfulness techniques, as well as to help implement actual mindfulness strategies within the healthcare system. The last set of scenarios offers an array of circumstances in medical education where mindfulness techniques can be utilized.

Scenarios to Implement Mindfulness in Healthcare

Stage 1: Initial Stress Arousal

- Scenario: Increased patient load in a general practitioner's clinic.
  - Mindfulness Technique: Preventative Approach.
  - Practice: A team meeting to discuss workload distribution, as well as when and how to implement mindfulness meditation stress reduction strategies for both providers and patients alike amidst a bustling office workflow. What resources can be used to provide guided meditations?
- Scenario: Long hours for medical residents leading to fatigue.
  - Mindfulness Technique: Resilience Building.
  - Practice: How and where to implement group meditation sessions to help manage stress and build emotional resilience in the morning and evenings. What resources can be used to provide guided meditations?

- Scenario: Nurses facing demanding shifts in a hospital ward.
  - Mindfulness Technique: Communication Enhancement.
  - Practice: How can a meditation practice, group or individual, be juxtaposed to a discussion between nurses in which concerns are expressed and support is being sought from each other. What resources can be used to provide guided meditations?

Stage 2: Persistent Signs and Compensatory Behavior

- Scenario: Emergency room team experiencing frequent interpersonal conflicts.
  - Mindfulness Technique: Communication enhancement.
  - Practice: How and where can regular conflict resolution workshops, implementing mindfulness meditation, be instituted into the workplace to focus on mindful communication and empathy. What would this workshop look like start to finish? What resources can be used to provide guided meditations?
- Scenario: High turnover in administrative staff at a healthcare facility.
  - Mindfulness Technique: Addressing systemic issues.
  - Practice: How can mindfulness meditation be included in a routine organizational review of work conditions and staff feedback sessions to identify systemic problems. What resources can be used to provide guided meditations?
- Scenario: Medical laboratory team showing signs of apathy toward work.
  - Mindfulness Technique: Preventative approach.
  - Practice: Introducing regular breaks with mindfulness exercises to prevent emotional exhaustion. Where can a safe space be designated for these breaks? What resources can be used to provide guided meditations?

Stage 3: Global Exhaustion and Disengagement

- Scenario: Oncology department experiencing high levels of burnout.
  - Mindfulness Technique: Resilience building.
  - Practice: Group therapy sessions for staff to build coping mechanisms and resilience. How and where can these sessions be built into the workflow and work space? What resources can be used to provide guided meditations?
- Scenario: Radiology team feeling disconnected and unmotivated.
  - Mindfulness Technique: Addressing systemic issues.
  - Practice: Revisiting team goals and values through facilitated workshops incorporating mindfulness meditation, with the goal of aligning individual and organizational objectives. What would this workshop look like start to finish? What resources can be used to provide guided meditations?

- Scenario: Administrative team at a hospital experiencing poor job satisfaction.
  - Mindfulness Technique: Communication enhancement.
  - Practice: Regular team-building activities incorporating mindfulness meditation to enhance interpersonal relationships and communication. How and where can these activities be conducted? What resources can be used to provide guided meditations?

Across Stages

- Scenario: Primary care team facing challenges in adapting to a new EHR system.
  - Mindfulness Technique: Preventative approach.
  - Practice: Stress management techniques including mindfulness meditation leading up to, immediately before, and immediately after the implementation of the new system. How can users be directed to a meditation before and after their training? What resources can be used to provide guided meditations?
- Scenario: Surgical team feeling the strain of back-to-back surgeries.
  - Mindfulness Technique: Resilience building.
  - Practice: Post-surgery debriefs implementing a pre-debrief mindfulness meditation, focusing on collective achievements and strengths while employing mindful breathing and listening, reinforcing a sense of individual and team accomplishment. The debrief can also be concluded with a brief group or individual meditation. What resources can be used to provide guided meditations?
- Scenario: Executive board at a top hospital dealing with strategic planning stress.
  - Mindfulness Technique: Addressing systemic issues.
  - Practice: Leadership mindfulness retreats focusing on mindfulness meditation to enhance decision-making capabilities and address systemic challenges. What resources, including mindfulness instructors, can be used to provide guided meditations during the retreat?

Scenarios to Implement Mindfulness with DEI

- Scenario: Medical School—Diversity Challenge
  - Context: Medical students from diverse backgrounds feel marginalized in class discussions.
  - Practice: Incorporating mindfulness can enhance empathy among students and faculty, encouraging more inclusive dialogues. How can mindfulness training workshops be integrated into the curriculum to foster a deeper under-

standing of diverse perspectives? What resources can be used to provide guided meditations?

- Scenario: Clinician's Office—Equity Challenge
  - Context: Patients from minority groups feeling their concerns are not taken seriously.
  - Practice: Teaching the office that clinicians practicing mindfulness can manage their own biases and reactions, ensuring equitable treatment. How can office leaders model this behavior and encourage staff to participate in regular mindfulness training? What resources can be offered to the hospital staff to entrain meditation long term?

- Scenario: Hospital Board Meeting—Inclusion Challenge
  - Context: Decisions made without considering the impact on all staff members.
  - Practice: Board members can use mindfulness to become more self-aware and inclusive in decision-making. How can regular mindfulness practice be integrated into meetings to promote inclusive leadership? What resources can be used to provide guided meditations?

- Scenario: Nursing Staff—Diversity Challenge
  - Context: Nursing staff from different cultural backgrounds feel disconnected.
  - Practice: Mindfulness can help in understanding and appreciating cultural differences, enhancing teamwork. How can a more mindful environment be created in break rooms where staff can engage in mindfulness practices to foster this understanding?

- Scenario: Patient Interaction—Equity Challenge
  - Context: A patient with a disability feels their needs are not fully addressed.
  - Practice: Clinicians can use mindfulness to become aware of any unconscious biases and ensure equitable care. How can mindfulness techniques be integrated into patient interactions to help in understanding and addressing patients' unique needs?

- Scenario: Administrative Staff Meeting—Inclusion Challenge
  - Context: Staff feeling their voices are not heard in policy-making.
  - Practice: Leaders practicing mindfulness can facilitate more inclusive meetings, ensuring all voices are heard. How can mindfulness training be offered for leaders to help them to create a more inclusive culture? What resources can be used to provide long term, regular meditation training?

- Scenario: Health Policy Development—Diversity Challenge
  - Context: Policy developers overlooking the needs of diverse populations.
  - Practice: Mindfulness can help in understanding the diverse needs of the population. How can mindfulness training be provided to policymakers to ensure diverse needs are considered in policy development?

Appendix E

- Scenario: Community Health Outreach—Equity Challenge
  - Context: Community outreach programs not reaching or being implemented in all demographics equitably.
  - Practice: Mindfulness can help staff recognize and address any biases in service delivery. How can regular mindfulness practice be implemented during outreach delivery to ensure equitable community engagement? What resources can be used to provide guided meditations in an outreach setting?

- Scenario: Hospital Recruitment—Inclusion Challenge
  - Context: Recruitment processes that inadvertently exclude certain groups.
  - Practice: Mindfulness can help HR staff in being more inclusive and less reactive in their recruitment strategies. How can a more mindful environment be created during the recruitment processes to help in fostering inclusivity. What resources can be used to provide guided meditations during recruitment strategy meetings?

- Scenario: Medical Research Team—Diversity Challenge
  - Context: Research team lacks diverse perspectives, affecting the scope of research.
  - Practice: Mindfulness can help team members appreciate the value of diverse perspectives. How can mindfulness meditation be incorporated into meetings to ensure diverse views are considered in research? What resources can be used to provide guided meditations during research meetings?

- Scenario: Emergency Room Dynamics—Equity Challenge
  - Context: ER staff inadvertently prioritizing patients based on biases.
  - Practice: Mindfulness can help staff recognize and address their unconscious biases. How can ED leaders embrace mindfulness to help set the tone for equitable patient treatment? How can mindfulness techniques be incorporated into the triage process and what resources can be used to provide guided meditations in this setting?

- Scenario: Hospital Staff Training—Inclusion Challenge
  - Context: Training programs not inclusive of all learning styles and backgrounds.
  - Practice: Mindfulness can help trainers be more inclusive and adaptive. How can regular mindfulness practice be implemented among trainers to ensure all staff members feel included and valued? What resources can be used to provide guided meditations?

Scenarios to Implement Mindfulness within Medical Education

Utilize these insights and techniques to practice individual or group mindfulness meditation throughout your medical education journey.

- Medical School Lectures:
  - Implementation: Integration of mindfulness exercises at the start of lectures.
  - Insight: Improves focus and retention of complex medical concepts.
  - Technique: Brief guided meditation focusing on breath to center attention.

- Clinical Skills Training:
  - Implementation: Incorporating mindful communication exercises in patient simulations.
  - Insight: Enhances empathy and patient-provider communication skills.
  - Technique: Active mindful breathing and listening practice in role-play scenarios.

- Exam Preparations:
  - Implementation: Mindfulness workshops to manage exam stress.
  - Insight: Reduces anxiety, leading to improved performance.
  - Technique: Visualization and body-scan exercises for positive outcomes and stress reduction.

- Residency Rotations:
  - Implementation: Daily brief team mindfulness sessions before rounds.
  - Insight: Builds team cohesion and prepares for challenging patient interactions.
  - Technique: Group mindfulness meditations focusing on intention setting for the day.

- Surgical Training:
  - Implementation: Mindful movement practices to enhance focus and steadiness.
  - Insight: Improves precision and calmness during surgical procedures.
  - Technique: Tai Chi or yoga sessions in addition to regular meditation practice to enhance mind-body coordination.

- Difficult Patient Encounters in Clerkships:
  - Implementation: Reflective mindfulness practice post-encounter.
  - Insight: Promotes understanding and managing emotional reactions.
  - Technique: Journaling followed by a mindful meditative or contemplative session.

- Interdisciplinary Team Meetings:

Appendix E

- Implementation: Starting meetings with a mindfulness moment.
- Insight: Encourages presence and effective communication.
- Technique: A short group meditation with intent focused on collective goals.

- Research Project Stress:
  - Implementation: Mindfulness training for managing project deadlines.
  - Insight: Fosters balanced approach to work and reduces burnout.
  - Technique: Regular mindfulness breaks focusing on breath and presence.

- Networking and Professional Development Events:
  - Implementation: Mindful networking exercises.
  - Insight: Builds genuine connections and confidence.
  - Technique: Body-scan and mindful breathing exercises prior to event kick-off.

- Post-Call Debriefings:
  - Implementation: Mindful reflection sessions after long shifts.
  - Insight: Assists in processing experiences and preventing burnout.
  - Technique: Guided group discussions with a focus on mindful sharing.

- Board Exam Review Sessions:
  - Implementation: Integrating mindfulness into study groups.
  - Insight: Reduces stress and increases focus during intensive study.
  - Technique: Mindful study techniques and group meditation breaks.

- Hospital Administration Internships:
  - Implementation: Mindfulness-based leadership training incorporating medical trainees.
  - Insight: Enhances decision-making and empathetic leadership skills, which then reflects on the trainee population.
  - Technique: Leadership exercises focusing on mindful decision-making and employee well-being with reserved spaces for trainees, free-of-cost.

Index

A
Acceptance and commitment therapy (ACT), 69, 73, 74
Acceptance training, 52, 53
Acute emotional distress, 82
Adrenocorticotropic hormone (ACTH), 41
Age and income inequality, 170
Age-appropriate techniques, 71
AI-assisted mindfulness, 156
AI-enhanced mindfulness app, 156
Amygdala, 29, 33
Angular gyrus, 30, 34
Anterior cingulate cortex (ACC), 44, 45
Anxiety, 31, 86
Anxiety-related sensations, 82
Applied/hybrid mindfulness, 20–21
Art and science of meditative practice, 19
Artificial intelligence (AI), 22, 149, 154, 156, 168, 169
  chatbots, 162
  networks, 155
Attentional control, 40
Augmented reality (AR), 157
Autonomic nervous system (ANS), 41
Awareness, 13
Ayurvedic medicine, 149

B
Big data, 97
Body scan meditation, 82
Borderline personality disorder (BPD), 72, 73
Brain theory of meditation (BTM), 37
Breath and scanning tactics, 90
Breathing exercises, 89
Buddhist philosophy, 71
Bureaucratic burdens, 97–99, 112
Burnout, 101, 102, 114

C
Caregivers, 96
Central executive network (CEN), 35, 36, 54
Charting, 137
Chatbot, 156, 157
chatGPT, 155
Chemotherapy, 91
Chronic stress, 5, 41, 42
Cingulate gyrus, 29, 31
Clinical consultations, 94
Clinical procedures, 94
Cognitive behavioral therapy (CBT), 69, 71
Cognitive flexibility, 50
Cognitive mastery, 129
Commodification, 163
Communication skills training, 137
Compassionate care, 112
Compassionate fulfillment, 100
Computational models, 48
Consciousness, 14
Contemporary secular programming, 21
Corticotropin-releasing hormone (CRH), 41
Cortisol, 41, 42
COVID-19 pandemic, 96, 147, 170
Cultivating mindfulness, 15

Cultural/language adaptation, 157
Cutting-edge technologies, 168
Cynicism, 5

D
Daily medical mindfulness, 159
Data tracking, 158
Default mode network (DMN), 30, 33, 54
Dialectical behavior therapy (DBT), 69, 72–73
Digital detox, 153
Digital diet, 152
Digital hamster wheel, 148
Digitalization, 147
Digitally-assisted mindfulness, 162
Digital mindfulness, 148
Digital stress, 148
Digital workplace, 148
Dilemma, 2
Diversity, equity, and inclusion (DEI), 119–121
Doctor/patient relationship, 4–5
Dorsal attentional pathway, 38
Dysphoria, 31

E
Electroencephalography (EEG), 37
Electronic health records (EHRs), 97, 112, 149
Emergency calm, 160
Emotional exhaustion, 169
Empathy, 98, 121
Endoscopy, 90
Equanimity, 136
Explainability of AI, 154

F
Faculty training, 140–141
False altruism, 101
Five Facet mindfulness questionnaire (FFMQ), 143
fMRI-adapted stroop world-colour task model, 39
Focused attention, 40
Focused/concentrative meditation, 18
Fragmented systems of care, 170
Fronto-parietal control network (FPCN), 30
Functional magnetic resonance imaging (fMRI), 29, 37

G
Gamifying, 158
Gratitude and compassion meditation, 94
Groundbreaking therapies, 168
Guided mindfulness, 157

H
Healthcare teams
  "archetypal" character styles, 113
  burnout, 111, 114
  clinical competence, 113
  communication breakdowns, 110
  compassion, 114
  compassionate care, 112
  decreased job satisfaction, 111
  DEI, 119–121
  emotional stress, 114
  empathy, 114, 121
  implementation, 123–124
  lack of attentional focus, 110
  passive-aggressive, 117
  perspective-taking, 121
  reducing reactivity and conflict, 121
  retention, 111
  stages of burnout, 116
  workplace stress, 114
Healthcare training
  better communication and interaction, 130
  clinical training settings, 136–137
  empathy and compassion, 129, 130
  engagement in educational settings, 133–134
  enhancing interpersonal skills, 129
  faculty training, 140–141
  feedback, 143
  formal lectures and workshops, 132
  head, 129
  heart, 128
  intense learning process, 129
  internships, 134–135
  longitudinal studies, 144
  measuring effectiveness, 143–144
  Monash's mindfulness programming, 141–143
  nursing and allied professional programs, 139
  objective assessments, 143
  observational assessments, 143
  patient feedback, 144
  residency, 135
  satisfaction surveys, 144

Index   227

  sequential/longitudinal training
      programs, 132
  sharpening the message, 138–139
  voluntary/compulsory, 137–138
Health disparities, 1
Hemodialysis, 91
High-stress environments, 169
Hippocampus, 29, 33, 34
Hospital/healthcare system, 6–7
Hypothalamus, 29

I
Imaginal rehearsal therapy (IRT), 83
Imaging, 89
Individual burnout, 115
Individual clinical consultations, 80
Individual mindfulness programming, 127
Inferior parietal lobe, 34
Insula, 33
Insular cortex (insula), 45
Integrating mindfulness training, 136
Integration in daily life, 24
Intellectual fulfillment, 99
Intensive treatment programs, 67
Interoceptive awareness, 30

K
K-12 elementary, 131

L
Lateral temporal cortex, 34
Limbic system, 29, 31, 32
Loss of connectedness, 2

M
Magnetoencephalography (MEG), 48
Malpractice, 103–104
Media ecosystem, 2
Medial prefrontal cortex, 34
Medical knowledge, 168
Medical office and hospital, 6, 80
Medical office staff, 5
Medical professionals, 6
Medical training, 5
Medicine, 96
Meditation, 3, 24
Meditation instructors/programs, 68
Meditation practices, 20

Mental healthcare, 80
Mental health disorders, 53
Mental health professionals, 68
Metaverse, 157, 158
Mindful AI, 155–156
Mindful Attention Awareness Scale
    (MAAS), 143
Mindful awareness, 4, 70, 92
Mindful break, 159
Mindful breathing, 20, 81, 93
Mindful community, 161
Mindful DEI, 122
Mindful focus, 160
Mindful healthcare professional
  bureaucratic burdens, 97–99
  burnout, 96, 101, 102
  compassionate, 104
  compassionate fulfillment, 100
  doctor-patient relationship, 95
  emotional regulation, 105
  empathic care, 104
  intellectual fulfillment, 99
  malpractice, 103–104
  personal fulfillment, 100
  presence and awareness, 104
  resilience, 105
Mindful healthcare setting, 10
Mindful healthcare system, 117–119
Mindful leadership, 123
Mindful life practice, 23–25
Mindful movement, 21, 22, 25, 161
Mindfulness 101, 9
  applied/hybrid mindfulness, 20–21
  awareness, 13
  meditation, 15, 24
  mindful life practice, 23–25
  mindful movement, 21
  mindful technology, 22
  misconceptions, 14
  moment-to-moment, 13
  non-judgmental, 14
  setting conditions, 17–18
Mindfulness and anxiety disorders, 43
Mindfulness-based cognitive therapy (MBCT),
    42, 43, 46, 71, 72
Mindfulness-based mind fitness training
    (MMFT) program, 39
Mindfulness-based pain management
    (MBPM), 69, 71
Mindfulness-based practices, 4
Mindfulness-based stress reduction (MBSR),
    20, 28, 42, 43, 46, 69–71, 140

Mindfulness-informed treatment programs, 69, 74–75
Mindfulness in medicine, 12
Mindfulness meditation, 35
Mindfulness practices, 148
  acceptance training, 52, 53
  attentional networks, 38–39
  breathing, 81
  BTM, 37
  clinical procedures, 88–91
  in clinical setting, 10
  cultivating resilience, 50–51
  doctor/patient relationship, 4–5
  during the visit, 86, 87
  emotional impact, 88
  empathy and compassion, 51, 52
  gathering and directing, 82
  gratitude/compassion meditation, 83–85
  hospital/healthcare system, 6–7
  impact of, 40–44
  implementation, 91–94
  limbic system, 29, 31–33
  medical office, 6
  medical professionals, 6
  monitoring, 91–94
  neural networks, 33–36
  neuromodulation, 31–33
  neuroplasticity, 31
  physical and mental health, 54
  post-visit, 87, 88
  pre-visit mindfulness techniques, 84, 86
  rehearsal/ modeled visualization, 87
  research limitations, 48–49
  scanning, 81
  science of, 9
  systems and networks, 29
  and technology, 10
  training programs, 7–8
  visualization tactics, 85
  visualization techniques, 82
  vulnerable moments, 87
Mindfulness research, 49
Mindfulness tactics, 98, 130
Mindfulness training, 24, 29, 39, 75–76, 93, 117, 127
Mindful technology, 22
  artificial intelligence, 149, 154
  bookending, 151, 152
  catalyst for mindfulness, 148
  chatGPT, 155
  daily medical mindfulness, 159
  digital detox, 153
  digital diet, 152
  digital stress, 148
  EHRs, 149, 151
  emergency calm, 160
  fraudulent "use", 163
  mindful break, 159
  mindful community, 161
  mindful design, 148
  mindful focus, 160
  mindful movement, 161
  mindset and organizational culture, 148
  predictive analytics, 158
  privacy and security issues, 163
  real-time feedback and guidance, 157
Mindful trainee, 145
Mindful training, 145
Mixed reality (MR), 157
Moment-to-moment mindfulness, 13
Monash University, 141
Monash's mindfulness programming, 141–143

N
Natural language processing (NLP), 157
Neural networks, 33–36, 155
Neuroplasticity, 31
Nociceptors, 44
Non-judgmental mindfulness, 14
Nurse practitioners, 110
Nursing and allied professional programs, 139

O
Observational assessments, 143
Office-based care, 84
Open/monitoring meditation, 19
Oxytocin, 42

P
Pali/smriti, 28
Paradoxical nature of healthcare, 1
Paradoxical situation, 1
Parasympathetic nervous system (PNS), 41
Passive-aggressive, 117
Patanjali's Yoga Sutras, 28
Path forward, 8
Patient care events, 136
Patient-centered care, 1, 7, 125
Patient education, 167
Perfectionism, 99
Personal fulfillment, 100
Personalized mindfulness programming, 156
Phlebotomy, 88, 89

Physician assistants, 110
Political melodrama, 120
Posterior cingulate cortex (PCC), 34
Post-traumatic stress disorder (PTSD), 60
Prefrontal cortex (PFC), 29, 32, 44, 45
Preventive care, 2, 3
Primary suffering, 71
Progressive muscle relaxation (PMR), 15, 20
Psychiatric and substance use disorder, 67
Psychiatrists, 68
Psychologists, 68

Q
Qi Gong, 16, 21, 22, 123
Questionnaires, 143

R
Radiotherapy, 91
Recurrent depression, 43
Reductionism, 3
Reductionist model of healthcare, 3
Regular practice, 123
Relevance alert system, 34
Resilience, 50, 51, 125
Retreats, 20
Rounding, 136

S
Saccadic movements, 16
Salience network (SN), 34, 54
Scanning, 93
Secondary education, 131
Secondary suffering, 71
Self-awareness, 98, 121
Self-care and prevention, 2
Self-reflection, 121
Self-related processes, 30
Self-report surveys, 143
Shift changes, 137
Social workers, 68

Socratic learning, 131
Somatosensory cortex, 44
Spiritual context, 28
Stress and uncertainty, 4
Stress management, 125
Substance use recovery programs, 67
Supportive environment, 123
Sympathetic nervous system (SNS), 41

T
Tai Chi, 4, 16, 21, 22, 123
Team burnout, 109
Team dynamics, 113–114
Telehealth integration, 157
Telemedicine platforms, 149
Thalamus, 29
Traditional exercise, 27
Traditional movement practices, 21
Training programs, 7–8, 133
Trypanophobia, 89
12-step model, 68

U
Undergraduate education, 131

V
Value-based healthcare system, 3
Ventral attentional pathway, 38
Virtual reality (VR), 157, 162
Visualization, 94

W
Walking meditation, 16
Wearable health devices, 149
Western contexts, 28

Y
Yoga, 4, 16, 21, 22

GPSR Compliance

The European Union's (EU) General Product Safety Regulation (GPSR) is a set of rules that requires consumer products to be safe and our obligations to ensure this.

If you have any concerns about our products, you can contact us on ProductSafety@springernature.com

In case Publisher is established outside the EU, the EU authorized representative is:

Springer Nature Customer Service Center GmbH
Europaplatz 3
69115 Heidelberg, Germany

Batch number: 09397551

Printed by Printforce, the Netherlands